Neurodevelopmental Disabilities and Employment

This book provides a comprehensive curriculum on essential job-related social skills that will aid educators, job coaches, behavior specialists, behavior analysts, and other professionals to improve employment outcomes of individuals with autism spectrum disorder and other neurodevelopmental disabilities.

The curriculum guides instructors through an objective behavioral assessment of critical, social, and problem-solving skills, and provides a framework for identifying individualized, effective teaching strategies using a response-to-intervention approach. This book will present a vocational social skills curriculum that is divided into two parts: The Vocational Social Skills Assessment Protocol (VSSA) and the VSS Intervention Protocol (VSSI). Chapters explore skills such as conducting the VSSA and VSSI, collecting data for the VSSA, and interpreting VSSA and VSSI results.

With a focus on evidence-based interventions that may be practical for supervisors to implement on the job site, this curriculum is designed to foster positive relations in the workplace and promote long-term employment.

Dorothea C. Lerman, Ph.D., is a Professor of Behavior Analysis at the University of Houston – Clear Lake, where she directs the master's program in behavior analysis and serves as Director of the Center for Autism and Developmental Disabilities.

Neurodevelopmental Disabilities and Employment

Helping Learners Prepare for Social Demands in the Workplace

Dorothea C. Lerman

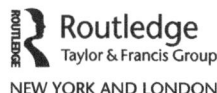
Routledge
Taylor & Francis Group

NEW YORK AND LONDON

Designed cover image: © Getty Images

First published 2023
by Routledge
605 Third Avenue, New York, NY 10158

and by Routledge
4 Park Square, Milton Park, Abingdon, Oxon, OX14 4RN

Routledge is an imprint of the Taylor & Francis Group, an informa business

ISBN: 978-1-032-31897-4 (hbk)
ISBN: 978-1-032-31892-9 (pbk)
ISBN: 978-1-003-31193-5 (ebk)

DOI: 10.4324/9781003311935

Typeset in Garamond
by MPS Limited, Dehradun

The book is dedicated to my husband, Robert Dempsey, who has spent the last 27 years anticipating my every need. To the moon and back.

Contents

Foreword

It is well established that many people with neurodevelopmental disabilities (NDD) often face obstacles in obtaining and maintaining successful employment due to challenges with social interactions in the workplace. This book is a treasure chest of practical information for helping individuals develop job-related social and problem-solving skills to overcome those challenges. The content centers on an assessment and intervention curriculum developed through the author's extensive research publications and experience in working with individuals with NDD in employment situations. The curriculum is described in step-by-step detail for assessing specific work-related social challenges on an individualized basis and then using evidence-based strategies to teach and otherwise promote specific skills to resolve those challenges.

The description of the curriculum is exemplary in its presentation. Numerous real-life examples are provided to illustrate the application of each curriculum component. Many working tools are likewise provided to facilitate the use of the curriculum in various social-related situations that are frequently challenging for individuals with NDD. Underlying all applications is attention directed to the employment and social preferences of individuals, and providing social-skill interventions that enhance access to those preferences. The concern for individual preferences, personally tailored assessment procedures, evidence-based interventions derived from the assessment, and data-based intervention refinement as needed make this book a gold standard for effectively supporting individuals with NDD in managing social challenges in the workplace.

Dennis H. Reid, Ph.D., BCBA-D

Acknowledgments

This book was not possible without the assistance of many colleagues and students. I am especially grateful to Charity English, Maggie McKinley, Nicole Lasserre, Dennis Reid, and Carson Whitford for their comments on earlier drafts of the book and to Carson Whitford and Charity English for their assistance in creating the numerous data collection forms and supplemental materials that appear in the appendices. A special thanks also goes to my colleagues Drs. Jennifer Fritz and Sarah Lechago, who, along with Amanda Davis, Megan Dora, Marisa Goodwin, Carolyn Grob, Justin Hunt, Channing Langlinais, Courtney Laudont, Kelsey Leadingham, Trena Rouse, Pia Som, Loukia Tsami, Natalie Villante, Bridgette White, and Daniel Wright, provided input and assistance in developing the protocols described in this book. I am particularly grateful to Dennis Reid, who inspired me to write this book and provided helpful tips and thoughtful support throughout the process. Finally, I am so appreciative of my mother, Roberta Lerman, who created the art below, and the illustrations that appear in Chapter 9.

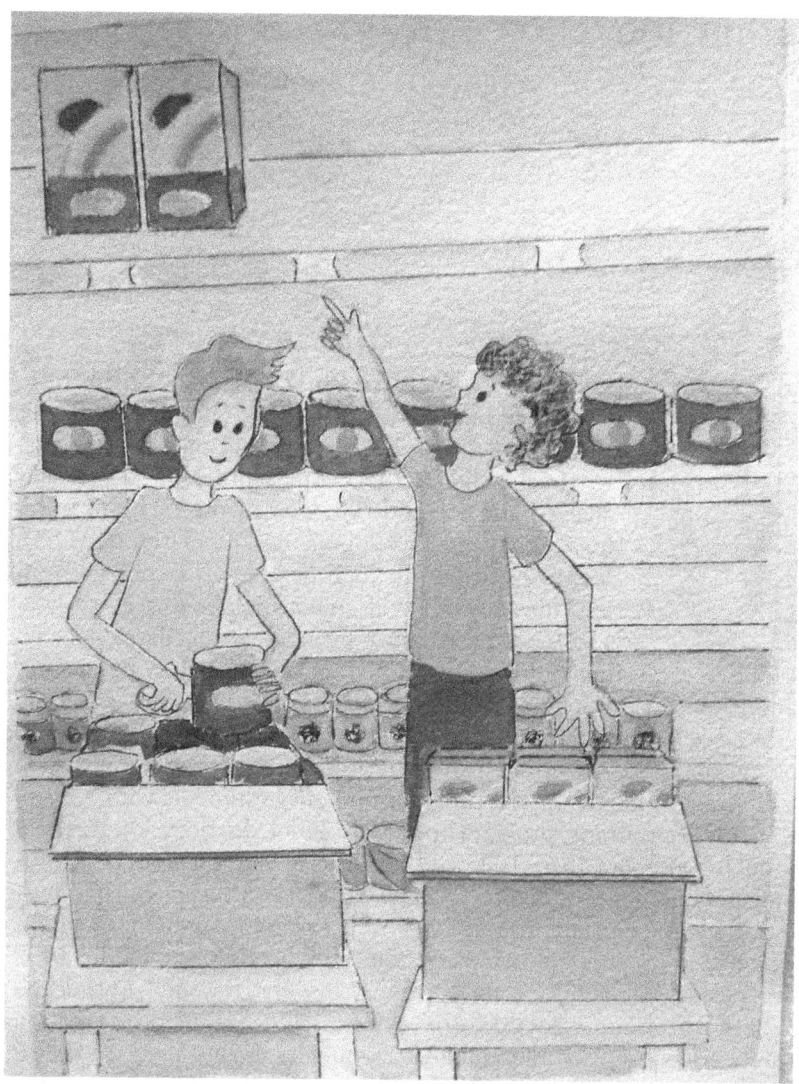

Illustration by Roberta Lerman. Used with permission of the artist.

Author bio

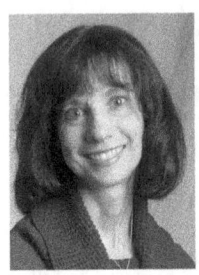 **Dorothea C. Lerman, Ph.D., BCBA-D, LBA-TX**
Dorothea Lerman is currently a Professor of Behavior Analysis at the University of Houston – Clear Lake, where she directs the master's program in behavior analysis and serves as Director of the UHCL Center for Autism and Developmental Disabilities (CADD). She received her doctoral degree in Psychology from the University of Florida, specializing in behavior analysis.

Her areas of expertise include autism, developmental disabilities, early intervention, functional analysis, teacher and parent training, and treatment of severe behavior disorders. She currently oversees several programs at CADD, including a focused intervention program for children with autism, a vocational program for adults with disabilities, a student support program for college students with autism, and a teacher training program for local school districts. Dr. Lerman has published more than 100 research articles and chapters, served as Editor-in-Chief for *The Journal of Applied Behavior Analysis* and *Behavior Analysis in Practice* and has secured more than $2 million in grants and contracts to support her work. She was the recipient of the 2007 Distinguished Contribution to Applied Behavioral Research Award and the 2001 B.F. Skinner Award for New Researchers, awarded by Division 25 of the American Psychological Association. She also was named a Fellow of the Association for Behavior Analysis-International in 2008. Dr. Lerman is a Licensed Behavior Analyst and a Board Certified Behavior Analyst.

1 Introduction

Why Focus on Employment?

Access to employment and other work-related experiences can greatly improve quality of life (Brand, 2015; García-Villamisar et al., 2002; McKee-Ryan et al., 2005; Taylor et al., 2014). Individuals who work are more likely to have adequate medical care and housing, have greater opportunities to develop social relationships, and are less likely to be dependent on others. However, successful employment requires a myriad of skills. To begin, the prospective employee must know how to search for available jobs, complete applications, and interview effectively. Once they have secured a job, the employee must complete assigned job responsibilities with a desired level of proficiency; follow directions; navigate the worksite; problem solve; interact effectively with supervisors, coworkers, and (possibly) customers; maintain good hygiene skills; manage their time appropriately, and ensure a reliable mode of transportation to and from work. And this list is not complete! This book primarily focuses on ways to build successful social relationships on the job.

Why Focus on Social and Communication Skills?

In light of the extensive list of competencies that are important for job success, why focus on job-related social-communication skills? First, employees frequently encounter situations that require good social and communication skills, such as asking for help when needed, responding appropriately to corrective feedback, making confirming statements when given instructions, and asking the supervisor for additional tasks when assigned tasks are completed (Montague & Lund, 2017; Partington & Mueller, 2015). Second, employers have repeatedly identified social skills as a high-priority area when surveyed about competencies that they value in their employees, with some even ranking this area above skills needed to effectively complete assigned job responsibilities.

Most importantly, employers have reported difficulties with social interactions as among the most common reasons employees lose their

DOI: 10.4324/9781003311935-1

jobs (Greenspan & Shoultz, 1981; Mueller, 1988). Consistent with these employer surveys, individuals with autism spectrum disorder (ASD) have reported difficulties interacting with supervisors and coworkers as among the top reasons they were unsuccessful with employment (Hurlbutt & Chalmers, 2004). My graduate students and I have assisted individuals who were fired for poor-quality work or off-task behavior because they would not ask for help when needed or locate other work to complete when their supervisors were unavailable. Other individuals were fired for insubordination after responding to feedback by arguing with supervisors and refusing to correct their work.

This research and our own experiences guided the selection of the specific social competencies included in this curriculum. Many of these social skills are critical to successful employment. However, other social skills can foster positive social relations between the employee and their supervisor(s), coworkers, and customers even though the skills may not directly impact whether the employee retains their job. Some examples of these additional "soft skills" include apologizing for mistakes, offering to help others when it appears needed, confirming understanding when receiving new instructions, and engaging in small talk with coworkers. By fostering good relationships, these skills may enhance the social benefits of working. Employers who have positive social interactions with an employee also may be more tolerant of social differences, more likely to overlook challenges, or more likely to give the employee the benefit of the doubt when issues arise.

Despite the importance of social skills for success on the job, these skills are easily overlooked among the myriad of competencies needed to obtain and maintain employment (Agran et al., 2016). Vocational training and rehabilitation programs often place greater emphasis on teaching individuals how to complete specific jobs rather than how to navigate the social challenges that arise in the workplace. Such an approach may lead to poor outcomes for those who find social situations particularly difficult.

Individuals with neurodevelopmental disabilities (NDD), including those with ASD, intellectual and developmental disabilities (IDD), and Attention-Deficit Hyperactivity Disorder (ADHD), may struggle with the social demands of employment. Indeed, there is growing recognition that problems with social-communication skills rather than with job-specific skills constitute the greatest barrier to employment success for individuals with ASD (Chen et al., 2015; Hendricks, 2010). One of the fastest-growing segments of those diagnosed with NDD, ASD is estimated to occur in more than 5 million people between the ages of 18 and 65 (~2% of the total population) in the United States (Dietz et al., 2020), yet less than 50% of adults with ASD have ever been employed and even fewer have full-time jobs (e.g., Barneveld et al., 2014; Burgess & Cimera, 2014; Shattuck et al., 2012; see also Chen et al., 2015, for a review).

Growing recognition of the dismal employment rate of individuals with NDD has resulted in a proliferation of organizations and service providers who are dedicated to helping them achieve success on the job. Those who support individuals with NDD, including educators, job coaches, vocational rehabilitation specialists, behavior specialists, behavior analysts, transition specialists, and other employment professionals, would benefit from a curriculum that focuses on essential job-related social skills, along with some associated problem-solving skills (e.g., what to do when your supervisor isn't available to help with a problem). A resource that would permit service providers to objectively evaluate a learner's current skills and to teach new skills using evidence-based strategies would promote their efficacy in helping this population obtain and maintain employment.

Focus on Replacement Behavior

This guide is intended to help professionals and caregivers improve the employment outcomes of individuals with NDD by targeting job-related social skills. It provides the tools needed to identify important social skills deficits and to develop effective interventions. To that end, this guide focuses on increasing appropriate social behavior rather than on reducing problematic reactions to challenging social situations. Professionals and caregivers commonly focus on problem behavior when they consider social barriers to employment. For example, we received a request to provide services to a young man named Samuel who tended to become argumentative when told to do a job differently, asked customers inappropriate questions, and refused to complete his work when given a new task. Consistent with the approach in this book, we did not directly target these inappropriate responses. Instead, we taught Samuel to emit the following specific socially appropriate responses in the relevant situations:

1 To thank his supervisor and confirm his understanding of the task when given corrective feedback,
2 To ask "How are you today?" and "Did you find everything that you need?" when greeting customers, and
3 To confirm his understanding of the task and his intention to complete it when given a new task.

That is, instead of arranging consequences to reduce inappropriate behavior, we taught Samuel what he should do when he encountered relevant social situations. The goal was for Samuel to engage in appropriate responses that would compete with, and thus replace, the inappropriate responses.

In many cases, teaching replacement behaviors is all that is needed to reduce problem behavior. For example, Mark, a 21-year-old man with

IDD, would often become argumentative and run away (i.e., elope) from the worksite when asked to do a task that was not typically part of his routine responsibilities. We hypothesized that Mark was attempting to escape these new tasks because he was not sure how to complete them. Rather than focusing on the argumentative statements and elopement, we taught Mark to emit a confirming statement and a request for help ("Ok, I will do the task, but can you show me how?") when he was given a new task. This statement effectively competed with argumentative statements by ensuring that the supervisor would show Mark how to do the task, thereby reducing the potential aversiveness of less familiar tasks.

The VSSA and VSSI

This book guides instructors through an objective behavioral assessment of critical social and problem-solving skills and provides a framework for identifying individualized, effective teaching strategies using a response-to-intervention approach. With a focus on evidence-based interventions that may be practical for supervisors to implement on the job site, this curriculum is designed to foster positive relations in the workplace and promote long-term employment.

This vocational social skills curriculum is divided into two parts: The Vocational Social Skills Assessment Protocol (VSSA) and the VSS Intervention Protocol (VSSI). The VSSA is designed to measure the performance of essential job-related social skills, along with other behaviors that may be critical for successful employment. In general, these social skills include the timeliness, frequency, and content of interactions between a prospective employee and other people in the workplace (i.e., supervisors, coworkers, customers). The assessment procedures can be implemented in a variety of settings, including actual jobsites as well as school-or clinic-based simulated work environments. The learner's behaviors are assessed by deliberately arranging social situations within the context of vocational tasks (e.g., arranging for the learner to run out of materials needed to complete a task). The results obtained from the VSSA depict current performance on social skills across a variety of vocational situations, along with key problem-solving skills and potential barriers to employment (e.g., problematic behavior).

As discussed in Chapter 2, *performance-based* assessments have a number of advantages over the more commonly used *indirect* assessments. Indirect assessments typically consist of surveys, interviews, and rating scales that are completed by a learner's caregivers, teachers, or others who are familiar with their performance. Yet, these assessments provide only limited information and have a number of disadvantages. For this reason, this curriculum emphasizes direct observation of performance and measurement of actual behavior in situations that arise on the job site. The VSSA

Protocol contains all materials necessary for preparing and conducting the assessment, collecting performance data, and reporting the results.

The VSS Intervention Protocol (VSSI) provides detailed, step-by-step guidance for selecting and identifying effective interventions for the targeted job-related social skills and for reducing barriers to success. The VSSI includes detailed descriptions of evidence-based interventions and instructions for evaluating their effectiveness via a hierarchical approach based on the relative intensity of the interventions. The goal is to identify the least intensive, effective intervention that would be practical for supervisors to implement on the job site. The VSSA and VSSI have been used primarily for the benefit of individuals diagnosed with NDD, but may apply to anyone seeking employment who may have deficits in job-related social skills.

What to Expect from this Book

This book is intended to serve as a curriculum and guide for professionals who would like to help prepare individuals with NDD for employment or assist those who are already employed but struggling with the social demands of the workplace. The intended beneficiaries of this book include educators, job coaches, vocational rehabilitation specialists, behavior specialists, behavior analysts, transition specialists, and other employment professionals. Further, the VSSA and VSSI protocols are designed for a variety of settings, including schools, training or therapy centers, and places of employment. For simplicity, the label "instructor" is used throughout this book to refer to the helping professional. The label "learner" refers to the various individuals who might benefit from these supports.

Chapter 2 provides an overview of the essential features of the VSSA and VSSI protocols. This is followed, in Chapter 3, by a brief primer on the basic concepts and procedures of applied behavior analysis (ABA), which serves as the basis for these protocols. Instructors with limited knowledge of ABA or those who would benefit from a review of ABA principles and procedures should find this primer helpful for understanding the interventions recommended in the VSSI protocol. All readers are strongly encouraged to review Chapter 3 prior to delving into the details of the VSSA and VSSI.

The remainder of the book is roughly divided into two parts. The first focuses on the VSSA. Chapter 4 describes all of the steps needed to prepare for and implement the assessment. Detailed instructions for collecting data on the learner's performance and for evaluating and presenting the VSSA outcomes are provided in Chapters 5 and 6. These chapters are accompanied by a number of forms, questionnaires, and data sheets that the reader can find in Appendices A and B. Across Chapters 4, 5, and 6, the reader is presented with a case example (John) to illustrate the preparation, implementation, and evaluation steps described in the VSSA protocol. Four additional case examples are provided in Chapter 7.

The remainder of the book focuses on the VSSI, with each chapter returning to John, the case example, to illustrate the process. Chapters 8 and 9 describe how to prepare for and implement the VSSI. Chapter 10 provides detailed recommendations for collecting data and monitoring performance during the VSSI, including the delicate process of making data-based decisions while evaluating the success of the intervention. Similar to the VSSA protocol, a number of accompanying sample data sheets and graphing templates are provided in Appendix B. Chapter 11 describes strategies for ensuring that the learner's performance maintains over time and transfers beyond the training setting. Finally, Chapter 12 returns to the four case examples introduced in Chapter 7. These case examples provide the reader with an in-depth look at how the VSSI might be applied across different types of learners, settings, and service modalities.

Should We Target This? Important Caveats to Consider

Before proceeding to the protocols, it is important to emphasize that just because a learner's social behaviors are *atypical* does not necessarily mean that they warrant intervention. On the contrary, interventions to create a more tolerant workplace are often key to the successful employment of neurodiverse individuals. The social behaviors included in these protocols were selected because of their potential to enhance relationships on the job. Depending on the features of the job setting and position, these behaviors may or may not be critical for the learner to maintain employment. Thus, although these protocols include behaviors such as making eye contact and conversing appropriately with coworkers, they should only be selected as targets after careful consideration of the learner's own desires and goals and the potential impact of these behaviors on the learner's employment. When considering a social target, it is important to ask two questions: Is this target critical to obtaining or maintaining employment? Is this something that the learner would like to target?

Box 1.1   Two questions to consider when selecting targets

1   Is this target critical to obtaining or maintaining employment?
2   Is this something that the learner would like to target?

Suppose, for example, a learner engages in self-stimulatory behavior (e.g., body rocking, finger-snapping) that is neither disruptive to the workplace nor will interfere with the learner's ability to complete their job responsibilities in a manner that is satisfactory to their supervisor. If the learner has no desire to change this behavior, it should not be targeted for intervention.

Ideally, the learner would value the skills that are needed to ensure their success on the job. However, as discussed later in the book, some learners may benefit from strategies to increase their motivation to learn new skills.

It is never too early to teach job-related social skills. For example, instructors of elementary school-aged learners can target how to respond appropriately to feedback and how to ask for help within the context of tasks and activities that occur at school or at home. However, it is also important to consider the pre-requisite skills that might be needed to effectively target job-related social skills. These will be discussed in Chapter 2.

References

Agran, M., Hughes, C., Thoma, C. A., & Scott, L. A. (2016). Employment social skills: What skills are really valued?. *Career Development and Transition for Exceptional Individuals*, *39*(2), 111–120.

Barneveld, P. S., Swaab, H., Fagel, S., Van Engeland, H., & de Sonneville, L. M. (2014). Quality of life: A case-controlled long-term follow-up study, comparing young high-functioning adults with autism spectrum disorders with adults with other psychiatric disorders diagnosed in childhood. *Comprehensive Psychiatry*, *55*(2), 302–310.

Brand, J. E. (2015). The far-reaching impact of job loss and unemployment. *Annual Review of Sociology*, *41*, 359–375.

Burgess, S., & Cimera, R. E. (2014). Employment outcomes of transition-aged adults with autism spectrum disorders: A state of the states report. *American Journal on Intellectual and Developmental Disabilities*, *119*(1), 64–83.

Chen, J. L., Leader, G., Sung, C., & Leahy, M. (2015). Trends in employment for individuals with autism spectrum disorder: A review of the research literature. *Review Journal of Autism and Developmental Disorders*, *2*(2), 115–127.

Dietz, P. M., Rose, C. E., McArthur, D., & Maenner, M. (2020). National and state estimates of adults with autism spectrum disorder. *Journal of Autism and Developmental Disorders*, *50*(12), 4258–4266.

García-Villamisar, D., Wehman, P., & Navarro, M. D. (2002). Changes in the quality of autistic people's life that work in supported and sheltered employment. A 5-year follow-up study. *Journal of Vocational Rehabilitation*, *17*(4), 309–312.

Greenspan, S., & Shoultz, B. (1981). Why mentally retarded adults lose their jobs: Social competence as a factor in work adjustment. *Applied Research in Mental Retardation*, *2*, 23–38.

Hendricks, D. (2010). Employment and adults with autism spectrum disorders: Challenges and strategies for success. *Journal of Vocational Rehabilitation*, *32*(2), 125–134.

Hurlbutt, K., & Chalmers, L. (2004). Employment and adults with Asperger syndrome. *Focus on Autism and Other Developmental Disabilities*, *19*(4), 215–222.

McKee-Ryan, F., Song, Z., Wanberg, C. R., & Kinicki, A. J. (2005). Psychological and physical well-being during unemployment: A meta-analytic study. *Journal of Applied Psychology, 90*(1), 53–76.

Montague, M., Lund, K., & Warner, C. (2017). *Job-related social skills: A curriculum.* 3rd ed. Reston, VA: Exceptional Innovations, Inc.

Mueller, H. H. (1988). Employer's reasons for terminating the employment of workers in entry-level jobs: Implications for workers with mental disabilities. *Canadian Journal of Rehabilitation, 1*(4), 233–240.

Partington, J. W., & Mueller, M. M. (2015). *The assessment of functional living skills vocational skills assessment protocol: An assessment, skills tracking system, and curriculum guide for skills that are essential for independence.* Pleasant Hill, CA: Behavior Analysts, Inc and Marietta, GA: Stimulus Publications.

Shattuck, P. T., Narendorf, S. C., Cooper, B., Sterzing, P. R., Wagner, M., & Taylor, J. L. (2012). Postsecondary education and employment among youth with an autism spectrum disorder. *Pediatrics, 129*(6), 1042–1049.

Taylor J. L., Smith L. E., & Mailick M. R. (2014). Engagement in vocational activities promotes behavioral development for adults with autism spectrum disorders. *Journal of Autism and Developmental Disorders, 44*(6), 1447–1460.

2 Overview of the Vocational Social Skills Assessment (VSSA) and the Vocational Social Skills Intervention (VSSI) Protocols

Key Features of the VSSA and VSSI

The VSSA and VSSI are designed to help providers and caregivers identify and improve social skills and related behaviors that may be critical for a learner's success on the job. These protocols are grounded in research and clinical experiences with a variety of neurodiverse individuals who desired to obtain and maintain employment. The protocols describe how to directly observe and measure performance during carefully arranged situations that are embedded within realistic work environments. The following sections describe key features of the VSSA and VSSI in greater detail.

Empirically Derived

The VSSA and VSSI, which are based on research conducted in my own clinical lab and by other scientists, draw from the literature on evidence-based practices in the field of applied behavior analysis. The VSSA protocol was developed and refined across approximately 10 years of clinical and research work (Grob et al., 2019; Lerman et al. 2017), during which my graduate students and I field-tested various versions of the protocol with more than 170 individuals. The VSSI protocol, which utilizes a response-to-intervention approach, also has been field-tested and researched in our clinical lab; however, the interventions draw from an expansive literature spanning more than 50 years that supports the efficacy of these practices (Heward et al., 2022).

Authentic Work Context

The goal of the VSSA and VSSI is to identify and improve specific job-related social skills while the learner is participating in authentic work situations rather than in role play or pretend instructor-led scenarios. The instructor can embed these protocols into any type of vocational

DOI: 10.4324/9781003311935-2

context, including school-, clinic-, or center-based simulated work or training programs; community-based work experiences; and paid employment.

The focus on realistic work situations is intended to improve the validity of the results and promote the transfer of skills from training to work environments. Because realistic work situations can be established in nearly any setting, many learners could potentially participate in and benefit from these protocols. Recent improvements in telehealth technologies also have enabled us to conduct the VSSA and VSSI remotely through the Internet, expanding access to the assessment and interventions described in these protocols. The case examples in Chapters 7 and 12 illustrate how the VSSA and VSSI can be conducted in a variety of settings and contexts, including those that must be supported through telehealth technologies (e.g., video conferencing).

Performance Based

The VSSA and VSSI are designed to measure the *performance* of job-related social skills and associated behaviors that will improve employment outcomes. As noted in Chapter 1, focusing on the learner's performance rather than on the learner's knowledge is the most direct way to identify and monitor acquired skills and skill deficits. It is entirely possible, for example, that a learner coulddescribe how they should respond when a supervisor gives them feedback. For example, they may say, "I should tell my supervisor that I will correct my work and then fix my mistakes." However, they may not behave appropriately when confronted with this situation. Conversely, a learner may be unable to vocally describe how an employee should respond when they are given a task that they don't know how to do. However, they may actually behave in an appropriate manner (i.e., ask the supervisor for help) when they are in this situation. As such, these protocols emphasize the actual performance of the selected social skills over the learner's knowledge or spoken descriptions of these skills.

Direct Observation and Measurement

As noted in Chapter 1, most commercially available social skills assessments rely on the reports of others to obtain information about the learner's skills and behavior. Caregivers, educators, and other professionals who are familiar with the learner may be asked to complete evaluative surveys, rating scales, and questionnaires about the learner's performance. Gaining information from informants about what they have observed in the past can be an efficient approach to assessment. However, research indicates that these types of *indirect assessments* can be highly unreliable and inaccurate. That is, what someone reports on a survey or questionnaire about what a learner can do may not closely match what the learner actually does in the relevant situation.

This disconnect is likely due to several factors. First, the informant may not have had sufficient opportunities to observe the learner in the relevant situations or contexts, possibly resulting in "best guesses" of how the learner might behave. These best guesses may be based on expectations or incomplete information about the learner's capabilities. For example, a parent or teacher may rarely observe how a learner responds in a certain situation (e.g., when given unclear instructions) if the situation rarely arises in the informant's presence. Indirect assessments also may be inaccurate because they depend on the informant's memories of past events involving the learner, some of which may be fairly remote. Finally, the accuracy of informant reports likely depends on the clarity of the questions on the surveys and questionnaires.

The most direct, accurate way to determine whether someone has a particular skill is to directly observe the individual and measure their performance in the relevant situations. Direct observation and measurement of performance are critical for both assessment and intervention. Measuring performance throughout the training process gives the instructor immediate feedback about the effectiveness of their intervention. These data permit instructors to continuously monitor outcomes, identify when the intervention is not working, and adjust their procedures as needed. Relatedly, this approach requires the instructor and learner to establish a goal level of performance for each targeted skill, commonly called the *mastery* criterion. This criterion provides a useful standard for determining whether a skill should be a target of intervention (based on performance during an initial assessment) and the point at which intervention should be considered successfully completed (based on performance during intervention). More information about measurement and data collection is described in Chapters 5 and 10.

Arrangement of Social Opportunities

Another key aspect of the VSSA and VSSI is the deliberate arrangement of situations that are relevant to the targeted social skills. The protocols specify exactly how to create these situations within the context of realistic work situations so that the instructor does not have to rely on naturally occurring opportunities to observe the selected social competencies. Directly manipulating relevant opportunities, or antecedents, enables a much more efficient assessment and intervention process. For example, suppose a provider is interested in observing how a learner responds when they encounter broken equipment that is needed to complete a task. The provider might have to observe for a lengthy period of time before the learner naturally encounters this situation in the work environment. However, the instructor could arrange for the learner to encounter broken equipment while working on relevant tasks. Controlling what occurs in the work environment permits the instructor to establish the desired number of opportunities to observe the targeted skills and for the learner to practice them as part of the intervention. Chapters 4 and 9 provide more detailed information about how to arrange these social opportunities, as well as how to respond to the learner's behavior during these encounters.

Individualization

Finally, the VSSA and VSSI provide the instructor with the flexibility to individualize plans for learners. Unlike many standard curricula, the protocols allow the instructor to select targets, goals, and interventions that are based on the learner's specific strengths, challenges, preferences, and learning history. The protocols also offer the instructor a variety of ways to track and monitor performance, ensuring that the data collection system meets the practical constraints of the teaching environment. Finally, the protocols can be implemented in a variety of settings and across different service delivery models. This latter feature is described in greater detail later in this chapter.

Scope of the VSSA and VSSI

As noted previously, the social situations and corresponding targeted skills selected for the VSSA and VSSI were drawn from both research and clinical experiences. The focus is on skills needed to be successful *once* employed rather than those needed to obtain employment (e.g., responding to interview questions from prospective employers). Social-communication competencies – even those that are most relevant to successful interactions on the job – are quite broad and would be difficult to completely capture within a single, comprehensive assessment. With that in mind, these protocols prioritize skills that are likely to build and maintain good social relations, solve problems, and compete with less desirable responses when a worker is confronted with situations that commonly arise on the job.

For example, one commonly occurring workplace situation that requires appropriate social interaction is when a worker needs assistance from a supervisor. Assistance may be needed in a variety of contexts, including when a worker does not understand task instructions or how to complete an assigned task, when a worker is unable to complete an assigned task because the necessary materials are missing or damaged, and when a worker completes a task and does not know what to do next. In all of these situations, the worker must recognize that assistance is needed, seek assistance in a timely manner, and interact with their supervisor in a manner that will resolve the problem and maintain good social relations.

It is also fairly common for workers to receive corrective feedback on the job or to be instructed to complete a task differently than before.

Responding to feedback in an unprofessional manner – a frequently reported problem – leads to poor employee-employer relationships and may be the sole reason for job termination. Some particularly challenging forms of feedback that employees sometimes encounter are those that include unclear instructions (e.g., "This is sloppy; please fix your work.") and directions that conflict with the original instructions. For a professional response, the worker should acknowledge the feedback, request clarification if needed, and correct the error without arguing or defending their work. More details about the specific targeted skills will be covered in Chapters 4 and 5.

The interventions included in the VSSI are based on the basic principles of applied behavior analysis (ABA) and have been studied extensively over the past 50 years. Furthermore, the protocol prioritizes interventions that are relatively efficient, low-cost, and nonintrusive; that on-site supervisors might be willing to implement; that focus on building appropriate replacement behaviors for inappropriate behavior; and that might promote the transfer of skills from training settings to actual job sites. These interventions can be applied when teaching any type of job-related skill, including those outside the scope of the protocols. The VSSI protocol recommends a unique response-to-intervention approach that permits instructors to develop individualized programs for their learners by identifying the necessary and sufficient level of intervention that will meet the learners' needs.

For example, the instructor might begin with behavior skills training (BST), which includes instructions, modeling, and roleplay. If the subsequent assessment indicates that the learner still does not perform the targeted social skill within authentic work situations, the instructor might introduce additional intervention components, such as on-the-job prompts and reinforcement.

This book is intended to be a useful resource for a variety of professionals, including those with limited knowledge of ABA. However, a basic understanding of key behavior-analytic concepts and terms is helpful to fully appreciate the recommended interventions and the reasons underlying their effectiveness with particular learners. To that end, a brief introduction to ABA is provided in Chapter 3 for those who may be less familiar with the field.

Prerequisites for Job-Related Social Skills

Although many learners can benefit from these protocols, it is important to consider the types of prerequisite skills that may increase the likelihood of success. It may be beneficial to target these skills first before proceeding with the VSSA and VSSI. One important consideration is the need to embed these protocols within the context of work situations. Thus, the learner should be able to complete at least some basic vocational tasks independently, such as sorting objects, folding paper or shirts, cleaning, or stapling papers. It is also helpful if the learner can remain on task without prompting for at least short periods of time (e.g., 10 min). This will enable the instructor to arrange opportunities for the learner to emit critical social skills (e.g., seek assistance when needed) within the context of authentic work environments (e.g., completing tasks without the supervisor in close proximity). As discussed more in Chapters 3 and 9, it is helpful if task completion or on-task behavior is maintained by some type of reinforcing consequence.

A second important consideration is the need for a functional form of communication. Regardless of whether the learner communicates via vocal speech, picture exchange, sign language, gestures, or a speech output device, the social skills targeted in the protocols require the learner to convey understandable messages to others. At a minimum, the learner should be able to emit a few requests and label a few items prior to targeting job-related social skills. When deciding whether to target social-communication skills with a learner who has minimal functional language, the instructor must remember that any interventions for social skills must include direct teaching of communicative responses that are not already in the learner's repertoire. The instructor will need to weigh the benefits of initiating social skills training immediately versus devoting time to building the prerequisite communication skills that will set them up for success. This consideration highlights the importance of starting early when teaching relevant social-communication skills.

Box 2.1   Prerequisites for job-related social skills

- Can complete a few basic work tasks independently.
- Has a functional form of communication.
- Can remain on-task for at least short periods without prompting.

Instructions for assessing and teaching these prerequisite skills are beyond the scope of this book. Resources for assessment of these skills include the *Assessment of Basic Learning and Language Skills (ABLLS®-R; Partington, 2010)*, the *Assessment of Functional Living Skills (AFLS®; Partington & Mueller, 2012)*, and the *Verbal Behavior-Milestones Assessment and Placement Program (VB-MAPP; Sundberg, 2008)*. Resources for teaching these skills include *Essential for Living* (McGreevy & Fry, 2014), *A Work in Progress* (Leaf, 1999), *Preference-Based Teaching: Helping People with Developmental Disabilities Enjoy Learning Without Problem Behavior*

(Reid & Green, 2005), and ABA textbooks, such as *Applied Behavior Analysis, 3rd ed* (Cooper et al., 2020).

Incorporating Protocols Into Current Service Delivery Models

Various professionals, including job coaches, vocational rehabilitation specialists, transition specialists, behavior analysts, and teachers, assist learners in acquiring vocational skills. These trainings occur in various settings, including therapeutic clinics, specialized training centers, schools, community businesses, and homes. Learners who participate in these services include those who are preparing for their first employment experience, those who have been previously employed either successfully or unsuccessfully, and those who are currently employed. All types of professionals can use these protocols with learners in various stages of the employment process, regardless of the service setting. This includes caregivers who are working with learners in the home environment. The following sections describe how these protocols might be arranged in the most common service delivery settings. Additional details about how the VSSA and VSSI can be implemented within the context of these settings are provided with the case examples in Chapters 7 and 12.

Therapeutic Clinics or Training Centers

Ideally, instructors in clinics and training centers can arrange the environment to simulate an authentic work setting by establishing designated areas for work, breaks, and the supervisor's office. The instructor also should establish a location for task materials and supplies, such as a cabinet or storage room. To observe performance within the context of different vocational settings, the instructor might set up multiple work areas by taking advantage of various pre-existing rooms, such as offices, bathrooms, mailrooms, and employee lounges. For example, an instructor could set up cleaning tasks in the employee lounge, kitchen, or restrooms; clerical tasks in shared offices; and stocking, inventory, or organizing tasks in supply closets or storage rooms. The case example named "Dayden" in Chapters 7 and 12 illustrates how services might be delivered in this setting.

Schools

The VSSA and VSSI can be conducted in the classroom or other areas of the school that afford opportunities for vocational training activities. In the classroom, the instructor might arrange different areas for work and breaks, or, if this is not possible, provide the vocational tasks at the learner's regularly assigned desk or workstation. Ideally, the instructor should establish a location for materials and supplies that the learner could access when needed. Many schools also arrange for learners to receive vocational training on campus but outside of the classroom. For example, students might clean the cafeteria or gymnasium, sell coffee to staff, organize and stock supplies in the school store, or assist staff in the school library or front office. Teachers working with students in these locations could incorporate the VSSA and VSSI into these regularly scheduled activities. The case example named "Sergio" in Chapters 7 and 12 illustrates how services might be delivered in this setting.

Community Businesses

The protocols can be embedded within a variety of different work experiences that occur in community settings. This includes training, volunteer, and paid work at local businesses and organizations. For example, school staff and vocational rehabilitation providers often partner with community businesses to provide vocational experiences for their learners. These business partners include large box stores, restaurants, grocery stores, thrift shops, animal shelters, and pharmacies. As part of these arrangements, the learner may sample a variety of jobs at a single location, obtain short-term work placements at several different businesses, or receive longer-term positions with companies that offer jobs matched to the learner's specific skills or interests. For example, at a pizza restaurant, the learner might assemble food take-out boxes, clean tables and floors, and stock supplies; at a large box store, they might clean restrooms, stock shelves, relocate returned items to the shelves, and return carts from the parking lot; at a thrift shop, they might fold and hang clothes, price items, and assist customers. Conducting the VSSA and VSSI within the context of these job placements is ideal because they offer an authentic work environment. However, it also requires the cooperation of the community site's staff, who likely will need to help the instructor arrange the situations necessary to observe targeted social and problem-solving skills. The case example named "Anika" in Chapters 7 and 12 illustrates how services might be delivered in this setting.

Homes

It may not always be possible to arrange simulated or authentic work situations in locations beyond the learner's residence. Even when a learner is receiving vocational training outside of the home, they may benefit from supplemental instruction. In such cases, in-home instructors or caregivers could arrange opportunities for the learner to engage in targeted social and problem-solving skills within the context of home-related tasks that also have relevance to some vocations. This includes tasks such as gardening and other yard work, cleaning the kitchen or bathrooms, doing laundry, and preparing food.

Virtual Modalities

Vocational services are not readily available to many families in this country. Families who live in rural areas or lack reliable forms of transportation may find it difficult to connect with relevant service providers. They may be unable to find any professionals in their area to provide the behavioral services described in this book. All of these barriers leave few alternatives for adult learners who no longer qualify for public education. An increasing number of health-related services are now available through virtual platforms. This may be one solution for learners who have difficulty accessing in-person vocational services. During the COVID-19 pandemic, we began to implement the VSSA and VSSI remotely through the videoconferencing platform Zoom. We have continued to offer services via this modality as we have found it beneficial for some families.

Families desiring these services will need access to a web-enabled device (ideally, a laptop or desktop computer), a camera, and a reliable Internet connection. With the assistance of family members, the instructor can arrange simulated work situations in the learners' homes by having the learner complete tasks in front of the camera while the instructor provides instructions and feedback via Zoom. Tasks that the learner can easily complete in this setting include folding and stapling papers, stuffing envelopes, folding clothes, sorting silverware and other objects, and completing computer-related tasks.

Prior to work sessions, family members can gather the necessary materials and make them accessible to the learner. For computer-related tasks, the instructor can send links to any needed materials via e-mail or the chat feature of the videoconferencing software and instruct the learner to share their screen so that the instructor can view the work. The instructor can observe how the learner performs without the continuous monitoring of a supervisor by muting their audio and video feed after giving the instructions for each task. More information about implementing the VSSA and VSSI using a virtual platform is provided with one of the case examples ("Michelle") appearing in Chapters 7 and 12.

References

Cooper, J. O., Heron, T. E., & Heward, W. L. (2020). *Applied behavior analysis,* 3rd ed . Hoboken, NJ: Pearson Education.

Grob, C. M., Lerman, D. C., Langlinais, C. A., & Villante, N. K. (2018). Assessing and teaching job-related social skills to adults with autism spectrum disorder. Journal of Applied Behavior Analysis, 52, 150–17210.1002/jaba.503.

Heward, W. L., Critchfield, T. S., Reed, D. D., Detrich, R., & Kimball, J. W. (2022). ABA from A to Z: Behavior science applied to 350 domains of socially significant behavior. *Perspectives on Behavior Science, 45,* 327–329.

Lerman, D. C., White, B., Grob, C., & Laudont, C. (2017). A clinic-based assessment for evaluating job-related social skills in adolescents and adults with Autism. Behavior Analysis in Practice, 10, 323–33610.1007/s40617-017-0177-9.

Leaf, R., McEachin, J., & Harsh, J. (1999). *A work in progress: Behavior management strategies and a curriculum for intensive behavioral treatment of autism.* New York: DRL Books.

McGreevy, P., Fry, T., & Cornwall, C. (2014). *Essential for living.* Orlando, FL: Patrick McGreevy, Ph.D., P.A. and Associates.

Partington, J. W. (2010). *The assessment of basic language and learning skills-revised* (ABLLS-R). Pleasant Hill, CA: Behavior Analysts, Inc.

Partington, J. W., & Mueller, M. M. (2012). *The assessment of functional living skills.* Behavior Analysts, Inc. & Stimulus Publications.

Reid, D. H., & Green, C. W. (2005). *Preference-based teaching: Helping people with developmental disabilities enjoy learning without problem behavior.* Habilitative Management Consultants, Inc.

Sundberg, M. L. (2008) *VB-MAPP Verbal behavior milestones assessment and placement program: A language and social skills assessment program for children with autism or other developmental disabilities: Guide.* AVB Press.

3 A Brief Applied Behavior Analysis (ABA) Primer

What is ABA?

Scholars and practitioners have been working in the field of applied behavior analysis (ABA) for more than 50 years. The goal of ABA is to improve behaviors that our society considers to be important. To do so, ABA focuses on observable behavior that can be repeatedly and objectively measured. The underlying assumption is that changes in the environment of the individual – specifically, events that occur immediately before the behavior and those that follow the behavior – are responsible for changes in behavior. Events that precede behavior, called antecedents, alter the likelihood that an individual will engage in a particular behavior at any given moment. Events that follow behavior, called consequences, alter the likelihood that the individual will engage in that behavior in the future. An individual's current behavioral repertoire is a direct result of their history with antecedents and consequences.

For example, when a tea kettle whistles (antecedent), an individual is likely to remove it from the burner and pour the water into their cup (behavior) because doing so produced a delicious cup of tea in the past (consequence). Related to job skills, when a worker is having difficulty completing a task (antecedent), they are likely to review available instructional materials (behavior) if doing so helped them complete tasks in the past (consequence). This is sometimes referred to as the "ABCs" of ABA.

Box 3.1 The "ABCs" of ABA

Antecedent →Behavior →Consequence

The approach underlying ABA is to modify relevant antecedents and consequences of a behavior to produce change (i.e., learning). *Behavior change* can include building new behaviors and strengthening or

DOI: 10.4324/9781003311935-3

weakening existing behaviors. The ABA approach to understanding and changing behavior is the same regardless of whether a behavior is desirable (e.g., thanking those who offer to help) or undesirable (e.g., arguing when given feedback).

Some Basic ABA Concepts and Procedures

This section provides a brief overview of some additional ABA concepts and their relevance to the strategies recommended in this book. Resources to consult for more in-depth descriptions of these concepts and procedures are provided in the reference list at the end of the chapter (Alberto & Troutman, 2012; Cooper et al., 2020; Mayer et al., 2022; Miltenberger, 2015).

Reinforcement

Reinforcement is an essential element of the ABA approach. Reinforcement is a consequence that increases the future likelihood of a behavior and ensures that the learner will continue to emit the behavior over time. For example, a worker will continue to ask their supervisor for extra breaks if the supervisor at least periodically grants the request (reinforcement). A worker will continue to complete their work on time if their supervisor regularly acknowledges their accomplishments (reinforcement). These consequences (extra breaks and supervisor acknowledgment) serve as reinforcers for the individual workers in these examples, but this isn't necessarily the case for all workers. It is important to identify the personal preferences (i.e., reinforcers) of individual workers when examining or modifying behavioral consequences. Some individuals might value attention from their supervisor or coworkers, whereas others might prefer to avoid social interactions. Table 3.1 lists examples of reinforcers that might be available in job settings.

Table 3.1 Examples of reinforcers

Food/drink
Videos
Music
Praise and other forms of attention
Positive performance evaluations
Additional or extra-long breaks
Assistance with tasks
Choice of tasks
Early dismissal or late start
Extra vacation days
Money, gift cards, tokens, and other types of conditioned (generalized) reinforcers

In general, reinforcement will be most effective if it occurs closely after the behavior. Supervisor acknowledgments, for example, may not reinforce behavior if they occur weeks or months after the employee has met their timeliness goals. If a behavior no longer receives any type of reinforcement, it is likely to decrease over time. This process is called **extinction**. For example, an employee will stop asking coworkers for assistance if they no longer offer the requested aid, and a supervisor might stop submitting paperwork early if they no longer receive positive performance evaluations for doing so. For this reason, it is important to ensure that reinforcement continues for any behaviors that are essential to success on the job. On the other hand, it can be helpful to withhold or minimize consequences that reinforce undesirable responses. For example, coworkers may need to stop providing aid to an employee whose requests for assistance are inappropriate (e.g., excessive).

The examples in Table 3.1 include reinforcers that others might arrange to help teach a learner new skills or to encourage a certain level of performance. This is referred to as **contrived reinforcement**. For example, a supervisor might give a worker extra compensation for completing tasks with a high degree of accuracy to encourage this level of quality. Alternatively, some behaviors receive reinforcement without someone deliberately arranging it. For example, coworkers may help an employee who requests their assistance. Although the assistance will serve to reinforce the learner's requests for help, the coworkers are not doing so to encourage this employee to ask for more help in the future. This is referred to as **natural reinforcement**.

Once a learner has acquired a skill or achieved the desired level of performance with contrived reinforcement, it is beneficial if the behavior receives natural reinforcement. The eventual goal is for the behavior to maintain with natural reinforcement only because this will increase the employee's independence on the job. To accomplish this outcome, a supervisor might gradually reduce contrived reinforcement after identifying effective natural reinforcers for the behavior. The importance of recognizing natural reinforcers for behaviors on the job site and strategies to reduce contrived reinforcement are discussed further in Chapters 9 and 11.

The examples in Table 3.1 also include stimuli that only function as reinforcers because they are associated with other reinforcers. Examples of these **conditioned**, or **generalized**, **reinforcers** include money, gift cards, and tokens. We only value these items because we can exchange them for things that we desire. As such, they will not be effective as reinforcers if the learner has little or no opportunity to exchange them for highly preferred items. Using these types of conditioned reinforcers is discussed further in Chapter 9.

Identifying individual preferences is critical when assisting others to be more successful on the job. Some people may highly value praise and money, whereas other people may most appreciate extra work breaks and the opportunity to work on their favorite tasks. As discussed in the next section, research has identified best practices for identifying individual preferences.

Natural reinforcers also come into play when considering the consequences that shape and maintain undesirable responses. Research has identified a number of common consequences that may reinforce inappropriate behavior. Referred to as the *function* of inappropriate behavior, these consequences can involve attention from others, escape from undesirable activities or events, and access to tangible items (see Box 3.2). In work settings, for example, people may respond to an employee's outbursts or refusals to work by providing a lot of attention (e.g., asking the employee to explain their behavior), by removing job assignments, or by giving them preferred items (e.g., leisure materials or beverages) in an attempt to calm the person down. If such consequences are reinforcing, the employee may continue to engage in those behaviors if they can access those reinforcers as a result. More information about identifying possible functions of inappropriate behavior is provided in Chapters 5 and 6.

Box 3.2   Common social functions of inappropriate behavior

- Attention From Others
- Escape From Undesirable Activities or Events
- Access To Preferred Items or Activities

Identifying Reinforcers

Research and practice in ABA have incorporated a number of methods for identifying an individual's reinforcers. Typically called **preference assessments**, these approaches incorporate both indirect and direct forms of assessments. Indirect assessments rely on questionnaires, checklists, and interviews that ask the learner to report on their likes and dislikes. Others who know or work with the learner (e.g., caregivers, teachers) also may be asked to report on the individual's preferences. An example questionnaire that can be completed by the learner or others is provided in Appendix A.

Although these questionnaires can be useful for identifying potential reinforcers in an efficient manner, they may not produce accurate results for everyone. Research indicates that for some individuals, direct assessments should supplement these reports of preferences. Direct assessments of preferences can be conducted in a variety of ways, but they all involve observing and measuring the individual's behavior with respect to potential reinforcers. For example, giving people opportunities to choose among a variety of items and keeping track of what they choose most often is an evidence-based approach for identifying reinforcers. Employers and instructors could easily implement this type of assessment by asking workers to pick what they would like to receive (e.g., gift card, early dismissal, a favorite snack in the break room) when they meet some type of goal. Detailed instructions and a data sheet for conducting an efficient preference assessment called "multiple stimulus without replacement" can be found in Appendix A.

As described previously, natural reinforcers also can maintain inappropriate behavior. Determining these reinforcers for individual learners can be useful for identifying and targeting appropriate replacement behaviors. A recommended method for identifying these reinforcers, called a *functional behavioral assessment*, will be discussed in Chapters 5 and 6.

Discriminative Stimuli

Certain events in the workplace will increase the likelihood that a behavior occurs. Called **discriminative stimuli,** they do so because, in the past, the behavior was reinforced in the presence of those events and not in their absence. In the example provided earlier in the chapter, the whistle of a tea kettle increased the likelihood that someone would pour water from the kettle into their teacup. As a discriminative stimulus, the whistle signals to the individual that they will receive a delicious cup of tea if they pour the water into their cup. The individual will receive a weak or tasteless beverage if they pour the water before the whistle has sounded.

Discriminative stimuli are important to consider when teaching job-related social and problem-solving skills because they help the learner perform the right behavior at the right time. For example, a worker is less likely to receive immediate assistance if they interrupt a supervisor's meeting to ask for help than if they wait until the supervisor is not engaged. The supervisor's availability is an important discriminative stimulus for the worker. As another example, a worker is more likely to receive positive attention and a new task assignment if they notify their supervisor when they have completed their job than if they wait until their supervisor notices that they are unengaged. Thus, a completed job is an important discriminative stimulus for notifying the supervisor and asking for a new assignment. Identifying the relevant discriminative stimuli for targeted behaviors is essential for both assessing and teaching new skills. For this reason, these discriminative stimuli are integrated into the arranged situations of the VSSA and VSSI, as discussed in Chapters 4, 8, and 9.

Prompts

Prompts are often indispensable for helping people perform the right behavior at the right time. Prompts can take a variety of forms. For example, in the presence of the relevant discriminative stimulus (e.g., a completed task), an instructor could provide a spoken prompt (e.g., "Tell your supervisor that you have finished with your work."), a gesture prompt (e.g., gesturing towards the supervisor's office), or a model prompt (e.g., demonstrating how to notify the supervisor of task completion). Prompts can also take the form of written instructions, scripts, and pictures that are available to assist learners when they encounter relevant discriminative stimuli. Prompts are a recommended component of the VSSI and will be discussed in greater detail in Chapters 9 and 11.

Motivating Operations

Like discriminative stimuli, motivating operations increase the likelihood that a behavior will occur. However, motivating operations do so by increasing the value of the reinforcer that typically follows the behavior. For example, water (reinforcer) will be more valuable to a worker when they are lifting heavy boxes on a hot day (motivating operation). Thus, a worker who is completing such a task will be more likely to emit behaviors that result in access to water, such as going to the water dispenser in the break room or retrieving a water bottle from their locker. Someone who works alone for an entire work shift (motivating operation) may find interactions with others (reinforcer) to be particularly desirable at the end of their shift. Thus, this worker may be more likely to seek out social interactions or respond positively to the social initiations of others after working alone for an extended period of time. Receiving a task that a worker does not know how to do (motivating operation) may increase the value of instructions for completing the task (reinforcer). When encountering such a situation, the worker may be more likely to ask the supervisor or coworkers for instructions or to search for available manuals or guides.

Like discriminative stimuli, identifying relevant motivating operations for targeted behaviors is critical when assessing and teaching new skills. As such they are also arranged during the VSSA and VSSI, as discussed in Chapters 4, 8, and 9.

Maintenance

The term **maintenance** refers to the continued performance of behavior over time, even after a portion or all aspects of an intervention have been withdrawn. For example, suppose an instructor uses prompts and reinforcement to teach a learner how to search for needed supplies. Once the learner consistently searches for supplies, the instructor systematically fades out the prompts and provides less reinforcement for correct responses. Yet, the learner continues to search for supplies, perhaps due to the periodic reinforcement arranged by the supervisor or the natural reinforcer of obtaining the supplies necessary for the job. Maintenance of skills enhances the employee's independence on the job and, thus, the likelihood of their success in this setting. Research has identified a number of ways to promote the long-term maintenance of behavior change. As discussed further in Chapter 11, the instructor can adopt a variety of these approaches within the context of the VSSI.

Generalization

The term **generalization** refers to the transfer of learning from a training setting or context to other settings, people, and situations. For example, suppose an instructor teaches a learner how to respond appropriately to feedback from their supervisor. The ultimate goal is for the learner to respond appropriately to feedback across different work sites, supervisors, and tasks without the need for additional training or support in those contexts. Like maintenance, the generalization of skills is critically important to successful employment. The instructor can integrate a variety of research-based strategies to promote generalization within the context of the VSSI, as discussed further in Chapter 11.

Shaping

A procedure called **shaping** involves reinforcing closer and closer approximations of a targeted skill until the learner engages in the desired behavior. Shaping is useful when teaching a skill that may be particularly difficult for a learner to acquire. The instructor starts by targeting an approximation of the behavior that the learner likely can easily master. Once the learner acquires the initial approximation, the instructor targets a closer, but likely obtainable, approximation. This process continues until the learner achieves the ultimate goal. For example, suppose that an instructor is teaching a learner with a very limited vocal language repertoire to notify their supervisor of task completion by saying the word, "Finished." The instructor might start by teaching the learner to say an approximation of "Finished," such as the sound of the initial letter F. Once the learner is consistently emitting this approximation, the instructor would teach the learner to vocalize a closer approximation, such as the syllable "fin." Additional successive approximations the instructor could target are the words "fini," "finish," and then finally, "finished."

Shaping also can be useful when modifying aspects of performance other than the response form. For example, suppose a learner's goal is to remain on-task for 30 minutes; however, they typically work for just 5 minutes prior to intervention. It might be particularly difficult for this learner to increase their time on task by such a substantial amount (25 minutes) as their first step. The instructor might set the learner's initial approximation at 7 minutes. The instructor then would continue to gradually increase the targeted time as long as the learner is successful.

Successful shaping requires careful planning before and throughout the teaching process. The instructor must identify the most appropriate initial approximation based on the current skills of the learner, determine the successive approximations that will help the learner reach their goal, and select criteria for transitioning from one approximation to the next during the shaping process. The resources listed at the end of the chapter should be consulted for more detailed guidance on shaping.

Chaining

Similar to shaping, **chaining** involves breaking a complex skill into smaller, more teachable units. Chaining is useful when the individual must complete multiple responses in a designated sequence to successfully perform a skill. For example, making a cup of coffee involves a chain of behaviors that might include (1) placing coffee grounds into the basket, (2) filling a carafe with water, (3) pouring water into the machine, (4) placing the pot on the burner, and (5) pressing the on switch. The response sequence is called a **behavior chain,** and the breakdown of component responses that make up a behavior chain is called a **task analysis.** For some learners, it is helpful if the instructor targets one response component at a time.

To teach a chain, the instructor might begin with the first step in the task analysis (e.g., placing coffee grounds in the basket). Once the learner has successfully acquired this step, the instructor would introduce the next step (e.g., filling a carafe with water). This process would continue until the learner can complete the entire behavior chain. It is important to emphasize that the component responses are not taught in isolation. As each new response is introduced into training, it is embedded within the currently targeted response sequence.

Many job-related social and problem-solving skills involve complex behavior chains. Table 3.2 displays example task analyses for skills that help employees successfully navigate two situations in the workplace – running out of materials needed to complete a task and discovering that the supervisor is unavailable to provide assistance. Breaking these skills into their component responses can help simplify the learning process.

Successful chaining not only requires the instructor to identify the component responses that underly a skill, but also the ideal order of these responses. The instructor should consider the current skills of the learner when determining how much to break down the skill into its component

Table 3.2 Example task analyses for social and problem-solving skills

When worker runs out of materials:	*When a supervisor is unavailable:*
1. Locate supply cabinet. 2. Look for needed materials. 3. If materials found in supply cabinet, bring them to the work area and complete work. 4. If materials are not located in the supply cabinet, search for the supervisor. 5. Determine if the supervisor is available. 6. Explain the problem to the supervisor. 7. Ask the supervisor for help in securing needed materials. 8. Bring materials to the work area and complete the work.	1. Return to work area. 2. Locate other work to complete. 3. Set a timer for 5 minutes. 4. Work until the timer sounds. 5. Repeat steps 1–5 until supervisor is available.

responses. For example, the first step of the task analysis for obtaining materials in Table 3.2 is "locate supply cabinet." Some learners may need to begin with an even smaller step, such as "walk to the storage room."

In addition to creating the task analysis, the instructor will need to decide whether to teach just one step at a time or multiple steps simultaneously. When teaching just one step at a time, the instructor must select a criterion for introducing each new step of the chain during the chaining process. For example, they might introduce a new step when the learner has correctly completed the previously introduced steps in the chain on three consecutive opportunities. For more detailed guidance on chaining, consult the textbooks in the reference list.

References

Alberto, P., & Troutman, A. C. (2012). *Applied behavior analysis for teachers*, 9th ed. Pearson.

Cooper, J. O., Heron, T. E., & Heward, W. L. (2020). *Applied behavior analysis*, 3rd ed. Pearson Education, Inc.

Mayer, G. R., Sulzer-Azaroff, S., & Wallace, M. D. (2022). *Behavior analysis for lasting change*, 5th ed. Sloan Publishing.

Miltenberger, R. G. (2015). *Behavior modification: Principles and procedures*, 6th ed. Cengage Learning.

4 Conducting the Vocational Social Skills Assessment (VSSA)

The VSSA Protocol

The purpose of the VSSA is to obtain a current "snapshot" of a learner's social-communication skills, along with associated work-related and problem-solving skills, across a variety of vocational situations. This information can be used to develop goals, individualize interventions, and monitor progress. The VSSA protocol is a handy tool for acquiring information about a learner's current skills at pivotal moments in their lives. Such pivotal moments might include the start of a new school year, the initiation of new vocational services, and entry into new training programs. At the same time, periodically repeating the VSSA can be useful for evaluating the outcomes of vocational services and training.

The VSSA protocol contains all information necessary for preparing and conducting the assessment, collecting performance data, analyzing the outcomes, and reporting the results. Although the protocol includes a variety of recommended arranged social situations and targeted responses, the VSSA can be adapted and individualized across learners. The following sections provide detailed guidelines for completing all steps of the VSSA and for tailoring the assessment to the learner's needs and goals. The chapter concludes with a case example.

Preparing for the Assessment

Initial Information Gathering

To prepare for the assessment, it is helpful to obtain the following information about an individual learner:

- Job preferences and goals
- Work tasks the learner already knows how to do (e.g., Can they sort items, fold papers?)
- Work tasks the learner does not know how to do (e.g., Can they count change, use Microsoft Excel?)

DOI: 10.4324/9781003311935-4

- Reading and writing levels of the learner
- Clock reading skills of the learner (i.e., Can they read analog/digital clocks, and keep track of time?)
- Forms (i.e. topographies) of potentially inappropriate behavior, situations that tend to trigger it, and ways that people often respond to it
- Prior job training and work experiences and any challenges encountered

Copies of the learner's individual education plans (IEP) or other psychological reports and assessments may assist in attaining this information when available. All other pertinent information may be obtained through direct observations or interviews with the learner, other services providers, and caregivers. A sample interview form to help guide this type of information gathering can be found in Appendix A.

Along with information about the learner, the instructor should gather as much information as possible about current or future job placements. This includes the responsibilities of employees in the targeted positions, characteristics of the work environment, and the expectations of supervisors regarding various social- and problem-solving skills. A sample interview/survey form for employers is provided in Appendix A.

Selecting Situations

It is recommended that most assessments include the situations shown in Table 4.1 because employees commonly encounter them in vocational settings, they require good social-communication and problem-solving

Table 4.1 Brief overview of recommended, arranged situations for the VSSA

Situation Name	Brief Description
Task Interrupted	The supervisor interrupts an ongoing task to ask the learner to switch to a different task that must be completed immediately.
Materials Needed	The learner encounters broken or missing materials or runs out of materials that are needed to complete a task.
Vague Instructions	The supervisor assigns a new task that can be completed multiple ways without clearly describing or demonstrating how to complete it.
Task Not In Repertoire	The supervisor asks the learner to complete a task that the learner does not know how to do.
Feedback Provided	The supervisor delivers corrective task feedback that is clear, vague, or conflicts with the original instructions.
Task Completed	The learner completes a task and does not know what to do next.
Supervisor Unavailable	The learner needs assistance, but the supervisor is unavailable.

skills, and they can be particularly challenging for many learners. Table 4.1 provides a brief overview of each situation. More detailed descriptions of each situation are provided later in this chapter.

The VSSA protocol includes some additional situations that instructors may want to consider for some learners, such as asking the learner to relay information to others, arranging for a coworker or supervisor to need assistance, assigning multiple tasks at a time to the learner, arranging for someone to compliment the learner, and asking the learner to return from a break at a designated time (or after a designated amount of time). Quick reference guides for including these situations in the VSSA are provided in Appendix A. Furthermore, the protocol provides guidelines for identifying and including other situations in the VSSA based on the information-gathering stage. Examples of this type of individualization are described in the case examples in Chapters 7 and 12.

One of the most important factors to consider when individualizing situations to include in the VSSA is whether the learner reportedly engages in inappropriate behavior. Within the context of employment, a behavior may be considered inappropriate if it would (a) introduce risks to the safety of the employee or others, (b) interfere with an employee's ability to do a job satisfactorily, (c) prevent others from completing their jobs satisfactorily, or (d) substantially reduce the quality of the employee's interactions with others. Such behaviors may range from engaging in inappropriate conversational topics to physically harming others.

Box 4.1   Considerations when determining whether a behavior would be problematic in the workplace

A behavior may be considered inappropriate in the workplace if it would

- Introduce risks to the safety of the employee or others.
- Interfere with an employee's ability to do a job satisfactorily.
- Prevent others from completing their jobs satisfactorily.
- Substantially reduce the quality of the employee's interactions with others.

After identifying potential inappropriate behaviors of a learner, the next step is to develop definitions of those behaviors for the purpose of observation and measurement during the VSSA. The instructor may need to ask the learner's caregivers, teachers, and other providers to describe what these behaviors look like. For example, a teacher may report that a learner often "picks on" other students. Asking the teacher to describe this behavior in more detail might reveal that the learner will take others' work materials, snacks, and belongings without permission. Additional guidance for defining behaviors is provided in Chapter 5.

It is then important to gather information about when and where the inappropriate behavior(s) typically occur. For example, if a learner reportedly engages in disruptive behavior (throws work materials, leaves the work area) when told to do multiple tasks at a time or to finish their work more quickly, the instructor should consider arranging these situations during the VSSA. Doing so will allow the instructor to verify informant reports, directly observe situations that may be particularly problematic for the learner, and gain insight into the types of social skills that could be targeted to replace the inappropriate behavior. The sample interview form in Appendix A includes a section to help guide information-gathering on inappropriate behavior. The case example at the end of this chapter and the cases in Chapter 7 illustrate this process in greater detail.

Selecting Tasks

The instructor should consider the setting and goal of the assessment when selecting tasks for the VSSA. For example, if the learner is preparing for first-time employment, it might be appropriate to include tasks that are typically completed in entry-level jobs across several different industry areas. When the instructor is conducting the VSSA in a simulated work environment, tasks that are practical to arrange within the context of the current setting and resources will need to take priority. When possible, the instructor may find it beneficial to include tasks that relate to a learner's preferred and nonpreferred work environments, with the latter intended to assess how the learner responds when asked to complete nonpreferred tasks.

Suggested tasks that may be easy to arrange and are relevant to entry-level jobs in a number of different industry areas include folding clothes, rolling silverware into napkins, stapling paper, shredding paper, cutting, assembling boxes, filing documents, punching holes in paper, stocking items on shelves or in drawers, alphabetizing books, cleaning tables, vacuuming and sweeping, washing dishes, printing documents, typing documents, searching the internet for information, counting money, making change, completing inventory, sorting items, folding letters, stuffing envelopes, and addressing envelopes. A listing of possible tasks related to different industry areas can be found in Appendix A.

When a learner has already identified a prospective employer or the instructor is completing the assessment on an actual jobsite, the instructor should prioritize tasks that employees complete in that setting or that the employer might potentially assign to the learner. Indeed, assessing a learner's skills in an actual job setting allows for a competency-based preview of task completion in addition to a sample of their social-communication skills within the context of that work environment. For example, common responsibilities in large box stores include stocking shelves, sorting returned items, cleaning bathrooms, bagging purchases, and greeting customers.

Some of the "standard" situations arranged in the VSSA require the instructor to select particular types of tasks based on the skill set of the learner. This includes the task-not-in-repertoire situation and the vague-instructions situation. For the task-not-in-repertoire situation, the instructor should assign a task to the learner that requires a skill outside of the learner's current repertoire. For example, the instructor might ask the learner to open and print a Microsoft Word document or to calculate change if they know that the learner has not acquired these skills. They might also select a multiple-step task that includes steps that require skills that are within and outside the learner's skill repertoire.

The vague-instructions situation is closely related but distinctly different from the task-not-in-repertoire situation. For this situation, the instructor should select a task that could be completed correctly in multiple ways, depending on the preference or requirement of the particular employer or supervisor. For example, an employee might file or sort items along more than one dimension (e.g., sort items by color vs. shape; file letters by date vs. the sender's name), fold shirts in different ways, or roll silverware into napkins in different ways. The learner might know how to sort items, fold shirts, or roll silverware into napkins. However, if the instructor assigns this task for the first time by providing a general instruction (e.g., "Please sort these items." "Please fold these t-shirts") without clarifying the desired way of completing the task (either by describing or modeling how to do so), this situation requires a social response from the learner.

Although both the task-not-in-repertoire and vague-instructions situations both require the learner to request help from the instructor, the contexts have important differences. We have found that individuals who correctly ask for help when given a task that they don't know how to do may fail to do so when given vague instructions for a familiar task. For most of the remaining situations, the instructor should select tasks that the learner can likely complete with minimal instructions or modeling. The list of potential tasks provided in Appendix A also includes suggested situations that might be arranged when assigning those tasks.

Selecting the Task Amount

In addition to the types of tasks, the instructor will need to consider how much of each task to assign to the learner or how much time to allocate to a particular task based on the expected amount of time that the learner will need to complete it. Efficiency may be an important issue. As described in more detail later in the chapter, the instructor should include each of the arranged situations a minimum of three to five times within the learner's VSSA to obtain an adequate "snapshot" of their social-communication skills. In some cases, the instructor can arrange for a situation to occur multiple times while the learner is completing one particular task (e.g., the instructor could provide corrective feedback several times). However, many of the recommended situations are necessarily restricted to a single opportunity per task (e.g., the instructor can give a vague initial instruction only once per assignment, and the learner can only complete the task once per assignment). Thus, the assessment may require a noteworthy number of different task assignments. This could lead to a rather time-consuming, lengthy assessment if each task requires a substantial amount of time for the learner to complete.

Instructors can increase the efficiency of the VSSA by assigning tasks that the learner can complete fairly quickly. In our work, we aim for tasks that the learner can complete in no more than 10 to 15 minutes. To do so, we carefully control the number of task materials provided (e.g., an envelope-stuffing task may include just 20 letters and envelopes) or the scope of the task (e.g., a cleaning task may involve vacuuming a small room and wiping several tables) while still ensuring we can embed the situations of interest. It should be noted, however, that lengthier tasks may be desirable when embedding multiple situations within the context of a single task or when it is beneficial to assess the learner's performance in the context of more extensive task assignments.

In some cases, it may be appropriate to simply end an uncompleted task and transition to the next task assignment once the learner has an opportunity to respond to the arranged situation(s). An instructor typically might do this when arranging the task-not-in-repertoire situation, as the learner could require an extensive amount of time and guidance to successfully complete the task.

Arranging the Environment

The VSSA can be implemented in a variety of settings, but the particular setting may greatly impact how the instructor arranges the assessment environment. Regardless of the setting, it is recommended to have the following distinct areas within the VSSA environment:

Work location(s)

The instructor should arrange defined areas or rooms where the learner will complete the tasks assigned during the assessment. The work areas should contain materials and equipment needed to complete the planned assigned tasks. In addition, the instructor should ensure that the work location(s) include additional tasks that the learner could complete if the instructor is not available to assist when problems arise with the current task (i.e., "supervisor-unavailable" situation). In established work settings, the instructor should consider any potential advantages of modifying the existing work environment. In some cases, it may be beneficial to control the number of coworkers or distractions in the area to examine the impact of these variables on responding, particularly if the learner has a history of difficulty working with others or in the presence of distractions. For example, an instructor might arrange for a coworker to engage in non-work-related conversation or to ask the learner for help with their tasks.

Supply location

The instructor should arrange a designated location for supplies that the learner may need during the VSSA. The supply area, closet, or cabinet might be located within the work area(s) or in a distinctly different area. As noted previously, it is recommended that the VSSA include situations that require the learner to obtain additional materials or equipment when they are missing, broken, or of insufficient quantity while the learner is completing assigned tasks. The instructor should ensure that the supply location contains some of the materials or equipment that will be needed. During some tasks, the learner should be able to locate and obtain those materials on their own; for other tasks, they will need to seek the instructor to request assistance.

If the VSSA is conducted in a real work environment that does not have an established supply location, the instructor should consider whether it is advantageous to modify the existing environment to include it. If the goal of the learner is to work successfully in that particular work environment and obtaining supplies is irrelevant to the targeted job(s), the instructor may opt to exclude this situation and the supply location from the VSSA.

Supervisor location

Ideally, the person who is serving as the "supervisor" during the VSSA will be located in a separate room or area that is distinct (and remote) from the work areas. Such an arrangement resembles many authentic work environments where the supervisor is not always in close proximity to employees. Positioning the supervisor in a separate room (i.e., office) provides an opportunity to observe whether the learner knocks on the door (if not fully ajar) and waits for an acknowledgment before entering the room. On the other hand, if the instructor is serving as the supervisor and is located remotely from the learner, they will find it more challenging to observe the learner in the work setting for the purpose of measuring performance. If possible, the instructor might recruit the assistance of another person to collect the performance data while the learner remains in their view or to serve as the supervisor while the instructor collects the data. In our own work, we have positioned cameras in the designated work and supervisor locations so that we can video record the VSSA sessions for the purpose of collecting performance data. This option, which may not be possible in all settings, requires the prior consent of the learner and anyone else who may appear in the videos.

When the VSSA is conducted in a real work environment, the instructor should consider whether it is advantageous to modify the existing supervisor's location. In some work settings, the supervisor might typically remain in very close proximity to their employees. Thus, if the goal of the learner is to work successfully in a particular work environment, the VSSA environment should resemble that of the desired setting.

Break area

The instructor can observe a number of important social and problem-solving skills by arranging a distinct break area that is separate from the work and supervisor locations and providing the learner with regularly scheduled breaks (e.g., 10 minutes every 2 to 3 hours) throughout the VSSA. Ideally, the learner should be able to access preferred activities, interact with other coworkers, and monitor time during breaks. More details about arranging the break situation and the types of behaviors that the instructor might measure are provided later in the chapter.

Developing the Assessment Plan

Prior to conducting the VSSA with a learner, the instructor should complete an assessment plan. The assessment plan summarizes the tasks, situations, and materials that will be included in the VSSA. The additional time needed to complete this plan is a worthwhile investment. Having a predetermined plan helps to ensure a smooth assessment process, as the instructor will need to set up each situation and arrange the associated task materials within the ongoing context of the VSSA. A predetermined plan also increases the likelihood that the VSSA will include all desired situations an adequate number of times. It is recommended that the instructor has an opportunity to observe and record all targets at least three to five times during the assessment.

The example assessment plan in Table 4.2 shows the flow and order of assigned tasks with the associated arranged situation(s) and materials needed to complete the tasks. This is a partial plan, showing just the first 9 sessions of a VSSA. In general, a single task will appear in each row of the plan, along with one or more planned situations and the materials needed for the tasks. The number of materials is indicated in the "materials needed" column to specify the predetermined amount of each task. Information in the materials section also will specify if the instructor

Table 4.2 Example assessment plan (partial)

VSSA Plan

Session	Task(s)	Arranged Situation(s)	Materials Needed
1	Roll Silverware; File Letters	Task Interrupted	15 napkins; 15 forks; 15 knives; 15 spoons; 20 letters, file box
2	Staple Documents	Materials Needed (staples in supply cabinet); Task Completed	10 sets of documents; stapler with 5 staples
3	Fill Salt Shakers	Task Completed	10 salt shakers; jar of salt
4	File Documents	Vague Instructions; Clear Feedback; Task Completed	20 documents; filing folders
5	Create Excel Graph	Task Not In Repertoire	Computer; data
6	Organize Office Supply Bags	Supervisor Unavailable; Task Completed	5 bags; 5 pens; 5 highlighters; 5 pencils; 5 erasers
7	Break (with peer)	End of Break	Leisure materials
8	Fold Shirts	Conflicting Feedback; Task Completed	10 Shirts
9	Shred Documents	Materials Needed (working shredder with supervisor); Complimented; Task Completed	20 documents; broken shredder

plans to arrange missing, broken, or insufficient amount of materials. For example, if the instructor plans to arrange for the learner to run out of staplers during a stapling task, the plan will specify the number of papers to be stapled and the number of staples to include in the stapler, to ensure that the learner will receive an insufficient amount of staples. The plan also should indicate if the needed materials will be located in the supply area or must be obtained by requesting help from the supervisor.

Sometimes more than one assigned task may be listed in a single row of the "tasks" column. This is necessary when arranging a task-interrupted situation (see the first row of the example plan) or a multiple-task situation. Additional illustrative assessment plans are provided with the case example at the end of this chapter and the cases in Chapter 7. A blank template VSSA Plan is provided in Appendix A.

Conducting the Assessment

The instructor might complete the entire assessment plan during a single "work shift" or class period, or across multiple workdays or class periods, depending on the setting and time constraints. It is beneficial to distribute the assessment across multiple days if the learner is unfamiliar with the setting or the person serving as the supervisor. This permits the learner to acclimate to the setting and people in the new work environment, resulting in a more accurate snapshot of the learner's performance. The person designated as the supervisor will provide the learner with all instructions, task materials, and feedback throughout the assessment. More than one person can serve as the supervisor during the assessment if necessary. It might be particularly desirable to arrange this if the learner's goal is to work for a business where employees are commonly supervised by multiple people (e.g., large box stores or grocery stores).

If the work setting is new to the learner, the supervisor should provide a general description of the assessment plan (i.e., "I will be giving you a number of work tasks to see how you do.") before beginning the assessment. The instructor also should tell the learner to dress and behave as though they are on an actual job site if the assessment will be conducted within a simulated work environment.

Tables 4.3, 4.4, 4.5, 4.6, 4.7, and 4.8 provide quick reference descriptions of the "standard" (recommended) arranged situations that were outlined in Table 4.1. Example quick reference tables describing additional situations are provided in Appendix A. The top row of each table contains a description of how the supervisor should set up and end the situation. Regardless of the situation, the supervisor should respond as naturally as possible to the learner's responses. For example, the supervisor should provide assistance if the learner requests it or avoid extended small talk with the learner if such practices are typical on the learner's current or potential job site. The supervisor also should react to the

Table 4.3 Quick reference description of the task-interrupted situation

Task Interrupted		
Supervisor: Provide a task with clear instructions. Before the learner has completed the first task, present a second task and explain that it needs to be completed immediately (e.g., "I need to you to stop sorting for now and fold these napkins instead"). Ensure that the first task materials remain in the work area. End the situation when the learner has completed both tasks or stops working for more than 2 minutes.		
Learner Behavior	**Definition**	**Opportunities to Collect Data**
1 Completes New Task	Immediately completes the second task as instructed.	Any time the supervisor interrupts the learner and assigns a new task.
2 Returns to First Task or Asks Supervisor	Returns to work on first task or asks supervisor if they should finish the first task	Any time the learner works on a second task after a first task is interrupted.

Table 4.4 Quick reference description of the materials-needed situation

Materials Needed		
Supervisor: Provide broken or inadequate number of materials necessary for task completion. Additional materials may be placed in a designated supply location prior to the assessment or kept with the supervisor. End the situation if the learner does not obtain the necessary materials and stops working for more than 2 minutes.		
Learner Behavior	**Definition**	**Opportunities to Collect Data**
1 Searches for Materials	Begins searching for additional materials within an appropriate amount of time (e.g., 1 minute) by looking in the supply area(s).	When learner does not have materials necessary to complete the task and does not request them before the supervisor leaves the work area.
2 Finds Additional Materials	Finds the additional materials necessary to complete the task.	Any time the learner searches a supply location for additional materials and the materials are available in the supply location.
3 Seeks Assistance	Searches for the supervisor within an appropriate amount of time (e.g., 1 minute).	Any time the learner does not ask the supervisor for additional materials before the supervisor leaves the work area, and the learner does not find the materials on their own.
4 Makes Help Statement	Describes the problem or asks for assistance. Examples: "I ran out of staples." "Where can I find more envelopes?" "The printer isn't working, can you help me?" "I can't turn on the vacuum."	Any time the learner seeks assistance or the supervisor is located in the work area after the learner contacts missing/broken materials.

learner's undesirable behavior in the same way that people typically do (e.g., give the learner a break to calm down; ask them what is wrong; ignore the behavior). If the instructor is not certain how people typically respond to the learner's undesirable behavior, a good rule of thumb is to provide no visible reaction, if possible, during the assessment (i.e., simply continue with the current activities).

Table 4.5 Quick reference description of the feedback-provided situation

Feedback Provided
Supervisor: Give the learner task feedback directly related to the accuracy of their work. Task feedback should (a) clearly describe the problem and how to fix it ("Clear Feedback"), (b) include only general statements about accuracy with an instruction to fix the work ("Vague Feedback;" e.g., "You didn't do this correctly; please fix your work; "You didn't do this how I asked; do it again."), or (c) clearly describe the problem and how to fix it but the feedback contradicts the original instructions ("Conflicting Feedback;" e.g., the supervisor initially tells the learner not to seal the envelopes but then gives feedback that they should have done so.). If the learner does not fix their work, either end the situation or repeat the feedback to provide another opportunity for a correct response.

Learner Behavior	Definition	Opportunities to Collect Data
1 Acknowledges Feedback	Provides an acknowledging statement. Examples: "Thank you for telling me that." "Oh, I am sorry." "I misunderstood." "My mistake."	Any time supervisor provides feedback.
2 Asks for Clear Feedback	Asks for clarification or describes the problem. Examples: "How can I fix my work?" "Can you show me how to fix it?" "How?" "I don't understand what is wrong with my work."	Any time supervisor provides vague feedback.
3 Confirms Feedback	Acknowledges that they will fix mistake(s).	Any time supervisor provides feedback.
4 Corrects Mistake(s)	Fixes work.	Any time supervisor provides clear feedback.

The three columns below the top row in Tables 4.3, 4.4, 4.5, 4.6, 4.7, and 4.8 delineate the expected learner responses (left column), a definition of each response (middle column), and the opportunity to score whether or not the response occurred (right column). Guidelines for creating behavioral definitions for targeted responses are provided in Chapter 5. Also, as described in more detail in Chapter 5, the data collector may not have an opportunity to score some responses within an arranged situation.

It should be noted that some behavior descriptions include the phrase "within an appropriate amount of time." For example, in the materials-needed situation, the definition of "searches for materials" states, "begins searching for additional materials *within an appropriate amount of time* ... by looking in the supply area(s)." This phrase

Table 4.6 Quick reference description of the vague-instructions and task-not-in-repertoire situations

Vague Instructions OR Task-Not-in-Repertoire		
Supervisor: Provide incomplete and/or nonspecific instructions to complete a task that may be completed in different ways, or deliver clear instructions for tasks that are outside of the learner's repertoire. End the situation when the learner has completed the task or stops working for more than 2 minutes. Optional: Deliver feedback to combine this with the "feedback-provided" situation.		
Learner Behavior	**Definition**	**Opportunities to Collect Data**
1 Seeks Assistance	Searches for the supervisor within an appropriate amount of time (e.g., attempts to complete the work for no more than for 5 minutes).	Any time the supervisor provides vague instructions, or tasks outside of the learner's repertoire, and the learner does not ask the supervisor for help before the supervisor leaves the work area.
2 Makes Help Statement	Asks for clarification or describes the problem. Examples: "How should I fold the shirts?" "I don't know how to do this." "I have never used Excel® before."	Any time the supervisor provides vague instructions, or tasks outside of the learner's repertoire.

Table 4.7 Quick reference description of the task-completed situation

Task Completed		
Supervisor: Ensure that additional tasks are not present in the work area. Give the learner a task with clear instructions and do not state what they should do when they have completed the work. End the situation if the learner has completed the work and remains idle for more than 2 minutes.		
Learner Behavior	**Definition**	**Opportunities to Collect Data**
1 Seeks Assistance	Searches for the supervisor within an appropriate amount of time (e.g., 1 minute).	Any time the learner completes a task, regardless of whether the task was completed correctly.

(Continued)

Table 4.7 (Continued)

2 Makes Done Statement	States that they have completed the task. Examples: "I'm done," "I finished." "Here you go".	Any time the learner completes a task and either seeks out the supervisor or the supervisor is present in the work area.
3 Inquires about Next Task	Asks the supervisor what tasks they should complete next.	Any time the learner completes a task and either seeks out the supervisor or the supervisor is present in the work area.

Table 4.8 Quick reference description of the supervisor-unavailable situation

Supervisor Unavailable		
Supervisor: Ensure that additional tasks are present in the work area, preferably tasks that the learner has already completed during the assessment (and, thus, knows expectations). Arrange a situation during which the learner will need to seek out the supervisor (e.g., task completed, materials missing). Remain out of view (e.g., absent from the usual supervisor location and hidden in another area) or unavailable (e.g., in a meeting with someone or on the phone) until the learner has searched for the supervisor and had an opportunity to respond to this scenario. End the situation by returning to the work area/checking in with the learner if they do not complete the third step (search again for supervisor) within the designated amount of time.		
Learner Behavior	**Definition**	**Opportunities to Collect Data**
1 Returns to Work Area	Returns to the work area within an appropriate amount of time after seeking the supervisor.	Any time the learner seeks the supervisor, and the supervisor is absent or unavailable.
2 Begins Additional Task	Works on another task.	Any time the learner returns to the work area after seeking assistance from an unavailable supervisor and an additional task is available.
3 Seeks Out Supervisor	Searches again for supervisor after a designated time has passed (e.g., 5 minutes) or when the supervisor is available again.	Any time the learner returns to the work area after seeking assistance from an unavailable supervisor.

signifies that a variable range of intervals may be deemed acceptable for completing some behaviors. Suggested time intervals have been provided in these instances (e.g., 1 minute). However, these values should be modified to reflect the expectations for the particular learner in the current setting or when on future job sites.

Case Example

This section introduces a case example with descriptions of how an instructor completed all aspects of the assessment steps covered in this chapter with a learner named "John." Additional case examples are presented in Chapters 7 (assessment) and 12 (intervention). John was 22 years old and diagnosed with ASD and ADHD. He lived with his parents and older brother. He had a high school diploma and had received some community-based job experiences through his high school before graduating. John had requested job placement services through the local office of the state vocational rehabilitation agency, which, in turn, referred him to a therapy clinic for an assessment to determine his readiness for competitive employment. An instructor at the clinic, "Charise," was assigned to develop and implement the VSSA. She planned to conduct the VSSA in the clinic setting because John was not currently employed or working in a job setting.

Step 1: Gather Information

Charise began the process by conducting interviews with John, his mother, and a former teacher. These interviews revealed the following information that was pertinent to the VSSA:

- John would like to work as a disc jockey but he would also enjoy stocking and cleaning jobs. He is willing to consider any type of job because he is not entirely certain what he wants to do.
- John likes working with other people and has gotten along well with his teachers and classmates.
- John received some job training experience at a fast-food restaurant and a hotel. He cleaned trays and cleared tablesat the restaurant. He rolled silverware and filled salt and pepper shakers at the hotel. This was his favorite job.
- John's household chores include clearing the table after meals, vacuuming, making the bed, and folding laundry; he sometimes needs reminders to complete these tasks but can complete them accurately.
- John knows how to complete basic office tasks, such as folding papers, filing, stapling, and sorting objects. He does not know how to use a computer or count change. He can tell time using a digital clock.
- John reads on a 4th-grade level and writes on a 1st-grade level.

- While in school, John was sometimes noncompliant when his teachers asked him to complete tasks. He did not like to be told to hurry and would repeatedly say "wait a minute" when he did not want to do something. His teachers would typically respond to noncompliance by giving him encouraging statements and assistance (e.g., "You can do it! You are a fast worker. I will help you."), and John would eventually complete the assigned tasks. John is fairly compliant at home and rarely engages in any inappropriate behavior. Occasionally, he will yell and go to his room when his parents ask him to complete his chores (vacuuming, folding laundry).

Step 2: Select the Arranged Situations

Charise decided to include all seven situations outlined in this chapter, as the vocational counselor requested a comprehensive assessment to determine John's "job readiness" and his need for intervention services before she referred him to a job placement provider. Charise also decided to include some additional situations based on information obtained during the interviews. Although the vocational counselor had not yet identified potential work placements or jobs for John, he had prior experience working in a hotel and restaurant and indicated that he enjoyed those settings. Charise thought it was likely that workers in those settings would need to relay information to others, return from breaks on time, and complete multiple assigned tasks. Thus, she decided to include those situations in the VSSA, using the quick reference tables provided in Appendix A of this book.

In addition, John's former teacher had reported that John was sometimes noncompliant when he was asked to do tasks that he did not want to do, particularly when told to complete them in a limited amount of time. Charise thought that it was likely that John might be told to complete a task in a short amount of time when working at a busy restaurant or other retail business. As such, Charise decided to include a "time pressure" situation in John's VSSA. For this situation, Charise planned to have the supervisor tell John that he had only a short period of time to complete certain assigned tasks (e.g., "John, we need all of this silverware rolled before the next shift starts in 15 minutes."). She then needed to determine what responses might be appropriate when a worker experiences this type of time pressure. In light of reports that John might engage in inappropriate statements during this situation, Charise considered potential appropriate social responses that might replace (i.e., compete with) inappropriate behavior. For example, a worker might tell the supervisor that they are concerned about getting the work done in time, ask their supervisor if it is possible to get more time, or ask their supervisor if is it possible to get assistance with the task.

Charise also had to determine how the supervisor should react if John refused to complete the task or engaged in inappropriate statements.

Table 4.9 Quick reference table for a time-pressure situation

Time Pressure		
Supervisor: Assign a task that John knows how to do and that would take at least 15 minutes to complete if working at a rapid pace. Tell him that it must be completed in 10 or 15 minutes. Examples: "John, please roll all of this silverware before the next shift starts in 15 minutes." "We need you to vacuum this conference room before the next meeting in 15 minutes." "Someone is picking up these shirts in 10 minutes. Please fold them so that they are ready to go." If John refuses to complete the task, repeat the instructions one more time and then end the situation if he continues to refuse. Ignore all inappropriate statements.		
Learner Behavior	**Definition**	**Opportunities to Collect Data**
1 Seeks assistance	Searches for the supervisor before the requested completion time	Any time John does not ask for help before the supervisor leaves the work area.
2 Makes Help Statement	Accurately describes the problem or asks for assistance. Examples: "I may need more time to complete the work." "Is there someone who can assist me in folding shirts?"	Any time he is told that he has a limited amount of time to complete a task.

She thought it likely that his future supervisors would tell him again to complete the task and then, ultimately, assign it to someone else if John continues to refuse. Charise created Table 4.9 with instructions and targeted responses for this new situation. More information about how Charise collected data during this situation is provided in Chapter 5.

John's final list of arranged situations is displayed in Table 4.10.

Table 4.10 John's arranged situations for the VSSA

Task Interrupted
Materials Needed
Vague Instructions
Task Not in Repertoire
Provided Feedback (Clear, Conflicting)
Task Completed
Supervisor Unavailable
Relay Information
Multiple Tasks
Time Pressure
Breaks

Step 3: Select the Tasks

Charise considered several factors when selecting the tasks to include in the VSSA. First, Charise decided that it would be beneficial to select tasks common to entry-level jobs in at least several different industry areas because John was preparing for first-time employment and the vocational counselor was not yet certain what types of jobs they would pursue for John. Charise also wanted to include both preferred and nonpreferred tasks because his teachers and parents reported that he was sometimes noncompliant with tasks that he did not want to do.

In the initial interview, John indicated that he liked his job responsibilities at the hotel, where he rolled silverware and filled salt and pepper shakers. Although John could not identify his least preferred tasks, John's mother reported that he sometimes refused to vacuum and fold laundry. Charise also needed to consider tasks that would be appropriate for the vague-instructions and task-not-in-repertoire situations. Based on the initial interviews, Charise knew that John could complete a variety of cleaning tasks, fold papers, file, staple, and sort objects, among others things, but that he couldn't complete any computer-related tasks or count change. Filing, sorting, and folding clothes would be appropriate for vague instructions, as these tasks can be completed in a number of different ways. Making spreadsheets in Microsoft Excel, printing documents, and counting money would be appropriate when assigning tasks not in his repertoire. Finally, because Charise was conducting the assessment in a simulated work environment at her clinic, she had to

Table 4.11 Final list of tasks and potential arranged situations for John

Tasks	Potential Arranged Situations*
Shred	Task Interrupted, Task Completed
Stuff Envelopes	Task Interrupted, Task Completed
Staple	Task Interrupted, Materials Needed, Task Completed
Roll Silverware	Task Interrupted, Materials Needed, Task Completed
Clean Tables	Task Interrupted, Materials Needed, Task Completed
Fill Salt and Pepper Shakers	Task Interrupted, Materials Needed, Task Completed
File	Vague Instructions, Task Completed
Fold Clothes	Vague Instructions, Task Completed
Stock Shelves	Vague Instructions, Task Completed
Alphabetize Books	Vague Instructions, Task Completed
Sort Cards	Vague Instructions, Task Completed
Create a spreadsheet in Excel®	Task Not In Repertoire
Create a graph in Excel®	Task Not In Repertoire
Print Documents	Task Not In Repertoire
Count Money in Register	Task Not In Repertoire

* NOTES: The instructor can deliver a time-pressure statement prior to any task and provide feedback during any task; the supervisor can be unavailable for any situation requiring supervisor assistance.

consider tasks that would be practical to arrange in this setting and with her current resources. With these considerations in mind, Charise generated a list of tasks to include in her assessment plan.

Charise's final list of tasks and potential arranged situations appear in Table 4.11. Charise did not plan to have John finish any tasks that were not in his repertoire due to the extensive assistance he likely would need to complete them. If John correctly asked for help with these tasks, Charise said, "Thanks for asking but I'd like you to do something else now."

Step 4: Select the Task Amounts

Based on John's availability, Charise scheduled his VSSA to occur during two three-hour "work shifts," each occurring on separate days at her clinic (for a total of six hours). Further, because Charise wanted to obtain an adequate sample of John's social-communication and basic work skills while he completed a variety of entry-level tasks, she felt that efficiency was going to be very important. As such, she selected task amounts that she felt John could typically complete in no more than 10 to 15 minutes. However, she also knew that it might be important to see how he performed with lengthier tasks. Charise realized that she would have an opportunity to evaluate his performance with lengthier tasks when she arranged the multiple-task situation.

Step 5: Arrange the Environment

At her clinic, Charise had three available rooms that would be appropriate to designate as John's workroom, a break room, and the supervisor's office. The designated work room contained two tables, chairs, a supply cabinet, a computer with printer, and a file cabinet. The break room, located about 30 meters from the workroom, contained a couch, television, several chairs, an end table with magazines and books, and a large wall clock (combined digital and analog). The supervisor's office, located across the hall from the workroom, contained a desk, computer, file cabinet, chairs, and a cart for holding and organizing the selecting task materials.

Step 6: Create the Assessment Plan

Before beginning the VSSA, Charise created the assessment plan shown in Table 4.12 to help her stay organized and to ensure that she arranged three to five opportunities for John to experience each arranged situation. She also was careful to document when she planned to ask John to relay information to another staff person at the clinic, who would receive the information, and the message that she would ask John to relay. Additional assessment plans are provided for the case examples in Chapter 7.

Table 4.12 John's assessment plan

John's Assessment Plan

Session	Task(s)	Arranged Situation(s)	Materials Needed
First Work Shift			
1	Fill Salt and Pepper Shakers; Clean Tables	Multiple Task; Task Completed	20 shakers, boxes of salt and pepper; spray bottle, cloth
2	Fold Clothes	Time Pressure; Task Completed	20 shirts; 10 pants
3	Roll Silverware; Vacuum Room	Task Interrupted; Materials Needed (vacuum in supply cabinet); Task Completed	15 sets of silverware, 15 napkins
4	File Documents	Vague Instructions; Clear Feedback; Task Completed; Supervisor Unavailable	20 documents that can be filed by type or name; filing folders
5	Relay Information	Relay Information (to front office staff)	Attendance list
Break			
6	Create Excel Graph	Task Not In Repertoire; Supervisor Unavailable	Computer; data
7	Organize Office Supply Bags	Vague Instructions; Materials Needed (extra pens with supervisor); Task Completed	5 bags; 3 pens; 5 highlighters; 5 pencils; 5 erasers
8	Relay Information	Relay information (to Charise's assistant); Time Pressure;	Message – "Charise needs staff timesheets"
9	Fold Towels	Conflicting Feedback; Task Completed	25 towels

(Continued)

Table 4.12 (Continued)

John's Assessment Plan

Session	Task(s)	Arranged Situation(s)	Materials Needed
10	Shred Documents	Materials Needed (working shredder with supervisor); Task Completed	20 documents; broken shredder
Second Work Shift			
11	Roll Silverware; Shred	Multiple Task	15 sets of silverware, 15 napkins; stack of paper; shredder
12	Staple	Missing Materials (staples in cabinet); Task Completed	20 sets of papers, stapler with 5 staples
13	Relay Information	Relay Information (to the clinic social worker)	Message — "Charise will be leaving early today"
14	File Documents	Vague Instructions; Clear Feedback	30 papers that can be filed by name or color; file box
15	Print Documents	Task Not In Repertoire	Computer, printer, 5 files
Break			
16	Stuff envelopes;Shred	Task Interrupted; Task Completed	30 letters and envelopes; Stack of paper; shredder
17	Count Money in Register	Task Not In Repertoire; Supervisor Unavailable	Computer; data
18	Sweep Floor; Clean Tables; Remove Trash	Time Pressure; Multiple Task	Broom, dustpan, cleaning wipes, filled trash can
19	Roll Silverware	Missing Materials (napkins with supervisor); Task Completed	15 sets of silverware; 10 napkins

Step 7: Establish the Data Collection System

Once Charise had selected the situations and tasks, arranged her environment, and created her assessment plan, her next step was to ensure that she had an appropriate plan to collect data on John's performance during the VSSA. The next chapter provides an in-depth description of the data collection process and returns to this case example.

Step 8: Conduct the VSSA

After completing Step 7, Charise had everything that she needed to conduct the VSSA. At the start of each three-hour appointment, Charise showed John the location of the workroom, supply cabinet, supervisor's office, and break room. She then followed her VSSA plan and completed it in two appointments. The results of John's assessment are presented in Chapter 6.

5 Collecting Data for the Vocational Social Skills Assessment (VSSA)

Collecting objective, quantifiable data on the learner's performance during the VSSA is critical for summarizing and interpreting the results and for sharing the findings with the learner and others. This requires a plan for collecting these data in a practical and efficient manner. The VSSA protocol contains a recommended measurement system, including suggested definitions for potential social and problem-solving targets and approaches for collecting data on performance when the learner is completing tasks and encountering situations arranged during the VSSA, as described in Chapter 4. In this chapter, we provide a detailed description of this measurement system, with associated data sheets and guidelines for individualizing the system as needed.

One of the most important steps in setting up a data collection system is to establish clear and objective definitions of any job-related behaviors that the instructor plans to track during the assessment. Although the VSSA protocol contains suggested definitions for recommended social and problem-solving skills, the instructor is encouraged to individualize the desired responses and associated definitions based on what is most appropriate for their learners and the relevant job settings. With this in mind, the first section of this chapter provides guidelines and examples for creating behavioral definitions.

Guidelines for Defining Behavior

Creating operational definitions for social and problem-solving skills is important for collecting reliable, accurate data on performance and for determining exactly what is expected of the learner when encountering situations on the job. Operational definitions are clear, complete descriptions of responding that include only observable and measurable features of behavior. More specifically, good definitions have the following three key characteristics:

1 Objective: They include only physical, observable aspects of the behavior.

DOI: 10.4324/9781003311935-5

2 Clear: They are unambiguous so that anyone reading the definition understands what is expected and will collect data in the same way.

3 Complete: They include examples of the behavior as well as examples that should be excluded, if needed, from the definition.

Box 5.1 Characteristics of good behavioral definitions

Good definitions of behavior are:

Objective
Clear
Complete

Objective definitions focus on observable aspects of behavior so that accurate data collection doesn't depend on the subjective interpretations of others. Table 5.1 shows examples of objective and non-objective (i.e., subjective) descriptions of behavior.

The descriptions of behavior also should be as complete as possible and include examples that may need to be excluded from the definition. A behavior may be considered desirable or undesirable depending on the context under which it occurs. For example, yelling may be inappropriate in the work area but perfectly fine when engaged with others during reactional activities. Leaving the work area may be inappropriate when an employee is expected to assist customers but appropriate when it is time for a scheduled break. Other potential exclusions may be based on the intensity or frequency of the behavior. For example, asking for help is appropriate when an employee needs assistance to do a task correctly and timely but may be inappropriate if they frequently ask others to help them finish their assigned duties.

Table 5.1 Examples of objective and subjective descriptions of behavior

Objective	Subjective
The learner leaves the area without permission.	The learner is afraid.
The learner pounds their fist on the table and says, "no" or "not now."	The learner is upset and wants to get out of working.
The learner asks the supervisor how to do the task.	The learner is confused.
The learner lays their head on the table.	The learner is tired.
The learner says, "thank you," or "I appreciate that," or similar statement of gratitude.	The learner is grateful.

The following template may be useful when drafting behavioral definitions:

(Name of Behavior) occurs when the learner (insert objective description of the behavior with actions that can be observed and counted or measured), (under a certain context, if applicable). Data should not be collected if (list all exceptions when behavior exhibited is permitted given a different context).

For example, an instructor might create the following definitions:

Example 1: Matthew's refusals occur when he hides his eyes with his hands, shakes his head no, and leaves his work untouched for more than 3 minutes. Data on refusals should be collected only when work tasks have been presented either verbally or in an implied fashion (work materials placed in his work area). Refusals do not include when Matthew covers his eyes to rub them or when Matthew shakes his head or vocalizes no appropriately such as when given a choice.

Example 2: Trish engages in property destruction when she throws items more than 1 foot from herself, bangs her closed fists against surfaces, and/or when she rips materials with her hands. Property destruction may occur in all contexts throughout her workday. Throwing items when given permission or when using recreation equipment such as a ball as designed should not be counted as property destruction.

Instructors can determine whether a definition is objective, clear, and complete by asking someone else to read the definition and, if possible, to collect data on the learner's behavior at the same time as the instructor. The goal is for both observers to agree on the occurrence or non-occurrence of the behavior based on the created definition. If the instructor and their partner do not agree, they should discuss the reasons for their disagreement and modify the definition accordingly. A summary of guidelines for defining behaviors can be found in Appendix A.

Collecting Data on Performance

A large portion of the recommended measurement system is dedicated to recording the learner's response to the situations arranged during the VSSA. The next section of this chapter focuses on a data collection system for documenting performance during these situations. Following this section, additional data collection systems are provided for the purpose of collecting data on additional skills and behaviors that might be of interest, including inappropriate behavior, orienting towards conversation partners, and on-task behavior.

Responding to Arranged Situations

As outlined in Chapter 4, the instructor will arrange a variety of situations during the VSSA, with each providing an opportunity to examine the learner's response. Sometimes, relevant situations may arise naturally in the work setting. The focus is on documenting whether or not the learner responds to the situation in a manner that would seem most optimal for the workplace. These optimal responses are outlined in the arranged situations quick reference tables provided in Chapter 4 and in Appendix A. However, the instructor may need to modify these definitions to best fit the learner or their preferred workplace using the guidelines described earlier in the chapter. Case examples that include these types of adaptations are provided in Chapters 7 and 12.

The **Arranged Situations Data Sheet** is designed to record all data related to the learner's performance during situations of interest during the VSSA. Appendix B includes two variations of this form, one labeled "Sample" and the other labeled "Template." The sample data sheet is pre-filled with the "standard" (i.e., recommended) situations and associated responses that might be included in the VSSA. The template version contains no pre-filled situations or responses, enabling the instructor to individualize the assessment and data collection for each learner. The instructor should use the template data sheet to document the learner's performance when arranging situations that are not included on the sample data sheet or in the VSSA protocol.

The top portion of both data sheets, as illustrated in Figure 5.1, has spaces to record the learner's name, the date(s) of the assessment, the name(s) of the instructor(s) who are serving as the supervisor(s), and name(s) of the people who are recording the data.

The arranged situations and corresponding learner behaviors are organized into sections on the data sheet. The first row of each section contains boxes where the instructor can record the session number that is linked to the VSSA plan. The remaining rows list the possible learner responses for the arranged situation, with boxes to indicate whether the responses occurred each time an opportunity arose during the assessment. The data collector marks each box in the row with a "+" for a correct response and a "−" for an incorrect response. Each box in each row represents another opportunity for the learner to emit the response, which typically occurs when the instructor arranges the particular situation during the assessment. Each row contains enough boxes for the data collector to record the outcome of an arranged situation up to six times during an assessment. It is recommended that the learner have at least three opportunities to emit each target behavior during the complete assessment. Thus, a single data sheet typically should be adequate for a learner's assessment.

Learner:_____ Date_____ **Arranged Situations Data Sheet** Instructor: _____Data Collector_____

Figure 5.1 Top portion of data sheet.

Vague Instructions/Task Not In Repertoire

Session #	4	5	10	14	20		# correct	# of opp.	%
Seeks assistance	-	+	+	+	+				
Makes help statement	+	+	+	+	+				

Figure 5.2 Completed section of the sample Arranged Situations Data Sheet.

A completed section of the sample data sheet is illustrated in Figure 5.2. This example shows the learner's responses during the vague-instructions or task-not-in-repertoire situations. For either situation, the data collector has scored whether the learner (a) sought assistance in a timely manner and (b) emitted an appropriate help statement. Recommended criteria for scoring these two responses as correct can be found in the quick reference tables in Chapter 4.

A completed section of the task-completed situation on the data sheet is illustrated in Figure 5.3. For this situation, the data collector has scored whether the learner (a) sought assistance in a timely manner, (b) emitted an appropriate "done" statement, and (c) inquired about the next task. This particular section of the data sheet contains the most boxes in each row because many tasks assigned during an assessment might end with this situation. Thus, the instructor will have many opportunities to score what happens when the learner completes a task and does not know what to do next.

As described in Chapter 4, the instructor may arrange multiple situations within the context of single assigned tasks. If so, the data collector will need to score the learner's responses in more than one section of the data sheet while the learner is completing the task. For example, suppose the supervisor gives the learner a stapling task without clear instructions (i.e., vague instructions), does not provide an adequate number of staples for the task (i.e., materials needed), and also arranges to be unavailable if the learner seeks assistance (i.e., supervisor unavailable). This single stapling task will have three arranged situations and possibly a fourth (i.e., task completed) if the learner eventually acquires the staples needed. Figure 5.4 illustrates the relevant completed sections of the Arranged Situations Data Sheet for this example (shown as session #4 in each relevant section of the sheet).

During some situations, a learner may not have an opportunity to engage in a particular response that is listed on the situations data sheet. In these cases, the data collector should record "N" in the box next to the response. For example, this commonly arises during the materials-needed situation. As illustrated in the first column of Figure 5.5, the potential targeted responses are (a) searches for materials in a timely manner, (b) finds the materials, (c) seeks assistance, and (d) makes help statement.

Task Completed

Session #	2	3	4	6	7	8	11	12	15	17	18	20							# correct	# of opp	%
Seeks out supervisor	+	-	-	+	-	-	-	+	+	-	+	+									
Makes "done" statement	-	-	+	+	-	+	-	+	+	-	+	+									
Inquires/Begins new task	-	-	-	-	-	-	-	-	-	-	-	-									

Figure 5.3 Example data collected on the Arranged Situations Data Sheet for the task-completed situation.

Vague Instructions/Task Not In Repertoire

Task Interrupted

Session #					# correct	# of opp.	%
Completes new task							
Returns to initial task/Asks							

Session #	4				# correct	# of opp.	%
Seeks assistance	-						
Makes help statement	+						

Feedback Provided

Session #	Clear (C); Conflicting (F); Vague (V)				# correct	# of opp.	%
Acknowledges							
Asks for clear feedback							
Confirms understanding							
Corrects mistake/complies							

Materials Needed

Session #	4				# correct	# of opp.	%
Searches for materials	+						
Finds materials	+						
Seeks assistance	N						
Makes help statement	N						

Supervisor Unavailable

Session #	4				# correct	# of opp.	%
Returns to work area	+						
Begins additional task	-						
Seeks out supervisor	-						

End of Break

Session #					# correct	# of opp.	%
Resumes Work							

Figure 5.4 Example data collected on the Arranged Situations Data Sheet when arranging multiple situations.

Materials Needed

Session #	2	9	11				# correct	# of opp.	%
Searches for materials	N	+	+						
Finds materials	N	N	+						
Seeks assistance	N	-	N						
Makes help statement	+	+	N						

Figure 5.5 Example data collected for the "materials-needed" situation using the Arranged Situations Data Sheet.

If the learner immediately notices that they don't have adequate materials to complete the task (i.e., before the supervisor walks away) and points this out to the supervisor by describing the problem appropriately, then the learner does not have an opportunity to search for materials, find the materials, or seek assistance (a, b, and c, above). Instead, the learner emitted an appropriate help statement (d, above). As illustrated in the second column (labeled session 2) of Figure 5.5, the data collector would score "N" for searching, finding, and seeking, and a "+" for the remaining response.

Suppose the learner searches for the materials in the supply area but the materials are not available. In this case, the learner would not be able to find the materials on their own. As illustrated in the third column (labeled Session 9) of Figure 5.5, the data collector would score "+" for searching (a, above) but "N" for finding the materials (b, above) because they were not available to be found. Instead, the learner should seek assistance from the instructor and emit a help statement (c and d, above).

In a similar manner, if the learner searches the supply area and locates the needed material, there is no need for the learner to seek assistance from the instructor or emit a help statement. As illustrated in the fourth column (labeled session 11) of Figure 5.5, the data collector would score "+" for searching and finding and "N" for seeking assistance and emitting a help statement. Finally, the data collector should score "N" for finding the materials if the learner does not search the supply area (i.e., there is no opportunity to find them if they don't search the supply area).

Summarizing and analyzing the results of data recorded on the arranged situations sheet will be described in Chapter 6.

Other Job-Related Skills

Additional job-related skills that are not included on the situations data sheet may be important for successful employment. Instructors might find it beneficial to document performance in these areas. Some suggested targets include confirming understanding of instructions, orienting to-wards conversation partners, remaining on-task, and completing tasks accurately. Suggested definitions of these behaviors are as follows:

- **Confirming Statements**: The learner states that they understand the initial task instructions or repeats parts of the instruction delivered by the supervisor, even if in a question format, to confirm that they understand the task. Examples include saying "OK." "I got it!"
- **Orienting**: Learner's face is oriented toward the supervisor or other conversation partner during verbal exchanges, except when the learner is visually attending to relevant task materials (e.g., looking at task materials while the supervisor provides a model for completing the task).
- **Task Accuracy**: Learner completes the task as instructed when given clear instructions and all necessary materials, and the task is within the learner's repertoire.
- **On-Task:** Learner is orienting toward and/or manipulating materials in a manner necessary to complete the task when given clear instructions and all necessary materials, and the task is within the learner's repertoire.

However, this list of suggested targets is not exhaustive and could include other possible behaviors that may be selected for individual learners. Other possible targets will be listed later in the chapter and through the case examples in Chapters 7 and 12.

The data collector can use the ***Additional Behaviors Data Sheet*** to collect data on these behaviors throughout the VSSA. These additional behaviors can be monitored throughout the assessment or, if more convenient, during a portion of the assessment, such as during a sample of assigned tasks. Appendix B contains three variations of this sheet, labeled "Opportunity-Based," Frequency-Based," and "Interval-Based." These data sheets provide three different ways to collect data on behavior. The following are general descriptions of these recommended ways to collect data:

Opportunity-Based

For this format, the data collector scores whether or not the behavior occurred when the learner has an opportunity to engage in the behavior. This approach is ideal when the behavior can only occur in certain situations. For example, confirming statements can only occur when the supervisor delivers an instruction; orienting can only occur when the learner is interacting with someone else. By tracking the occurrence of those opportunities along with the behavior, the data collector obtains the most accurate picture of the learner's skills.

Frequency-Based

For this format, the data collector marks the data sheet each time the behavior occurs. This approach is ideal when the behavior is of short duration and can occur at any time during the VSSA. It also may be preferable when the behavior can occur multiple times during circumscribed opportunities. For example, inappropriate behavior can occur at any time (and multiple times) during work sessions. By tracking each occurrence of these behaviors, the data collector obtains a more complete picture of the learner's responses.

Interval-Based

This format is similar to opportunity-based recording but the "opportunities" are specific time periods of observing. The recommended interval-based recording is called "momentary time sampling." For this method, the data collector observes the learner at the end of designated time intervals (e.g., every 5 minutes) and records whether or not the learner is engaging in the targeted behavior. Interval-based recording may be a desirable alternative when frequency recording is neither practical nor appropriate. For example, this format may be ideal if the behavior occurs at high levels or the data collector cannot continuously observe the learner during work sessions. Interval-based recording also may be more appropriate than frequency recording when the targeted behavior is of long duration (e.g., on-task behavior). Research on this type of data collection system indicates that interval lengths of no more than 5 minutes will provide a reasonably accurate estimate of the true level of behavior.

Using the ***opportunity-based format*** of the ***Additional Behaviors Data Sheet*** to collect data on confirming statements is illustrated in Figure 5.6. The first and second rows include spaces to enter the date and consecutive number of each opportunity. In each box next to the behavior ("confirming statements") the data collector scores a "+" or a "–" to indicate whether or not the learner emits a confirming statement when the supervisor assigns a new task at the start of each session. The data sheet contains enough space to record the learner's response in up to 20 sessions. Depending on the number of tasks assigned during the assessment, it may be possible to capture all of the opportunities in a single data sheet for the assessment. A sample of responses to 20 opportunities may be adequate to estimate the current level of performance.

Example data collected for orienting using the ***opportunity-based format*** is illustrated in Figure 5.7. In each box, the data collector scores a "+" or a "–" to indicate whether or not the learner orients toward the speaker or listener (or provides eye contact, depending on the target) when the learner speaks to someone or someone speaks to the learner.

Opportunity-Based Recording

Scoring: (+) correct; (-) incorrect; On-task (+) scored if no more than _____ minutes/seconds off task

Date	6/1	6/1	6/1	6/4	6/5	6/5	6/5							# correct	# of opp.	%
Opportunities or Session #	1	2	3	4	5	6	7	8								
Confirming statements	+	+	-	+	-	-	-	+								

Figure 5.6 Example data collected for confirming statements using the opportunity-based format of the Additional Behaviors Data Sheet.

Scoring: (+) correct; (-) incorrect; On-task (+) scored if no more than _____ minutes/seconds off task

Date	6/1	6/1	6/1	6/4	6/4	6/5	6/5	6/5	6/6	6/6	6/7	6/7	6/7			# correct	# of opp.	%
Opportunities or Session #																		
Orienting	+	+	+	+	-	+	-	+	-	-	+	-	-					

Figure 5.7 Example data collected for orienting using the opportunity-based format of the Additional Behaviors Data Sheet.

Because these opportunities could occur multiple times within and across work sessions, the instructor does not record specific session numbers in the second row of the data sheet. The data sheet contains enough space to record up to 20 opportunities. It is highly likely that more than 20 opportunities will occur during a complete assessment, but a sample of 20 responses may be adequate to determine if this might be a target for intervention.

Example data collected for task accuracy using the ***opportunity-based format*** is illustrated in Figure 5.8. The opportunity to score whether or not the learner completed the task accurately is an assignment of a particular task that is within the learner's repertoire, and the learner is given clear instructions and all necessary materials (see suggested definition of task accuracy earlier in the chapter). To link the accuracy data to specific tasks, the data collector records the session number from the VSSA plan in the second row of the data sheet as an alternative to writing down the specific task. Below these session numbers, the data collector scores a "+" or a "–" in each box to indicate whether or not the learner completed the corresponding assigned task correctly.

In this example, the data collector is scoring task accuracy in an all-or-none manner, meaning that they only specify whether or not the learner completed the entire task correctly. This requires a criterion for correct completion of the task, which might be based on both the quantity and quality of the work (e.g., at least 90% of the silverware rolled correctly). For some learners, it might be desirable to collect more precise data on task accuracy. For example, it might be useful to document whether they completed the task with or without assistance (e.g., by recording the number or types of prompts required) or whether they completed certain aspects of the task correctly versus incorrectly (e.g., for an envelope stuffing task, noting that they inserted the letters correctly but failed to always seal the envelopes).

Example data collected for on-task behavior is illustrated in Figure 5.9. The opportunity to score on-task behavior is identical to that described previously for task accuracy. This format for on-task behavior using the ***opportunity-based format*** provides a relatively simple way to document on-task behavior while linking it to performance during specific tasks. This option might be desirable when a rough estimate of on-task behavior is appropriate, and when ease of recording is a priority over gaining more precise information about responding, such as the total amount of time that the learner remained on task. It requires the instructor to pre-specify the criteria for scoring the learner as either on-task or off-task while they are completing an assigned task. For example, the instructor might determine that a learner would be scored as "on task" as long as they did not stop working for more than 2 minutes during the assigned task. A more stringent criterion might require that the learner work continuously without stopping until they complete the

Scoring: (+) correct; (-) incorrect; On-task (+) scored if no more than _____ minutes/seconds off task:

Date	6/1	6/1	6/1	6/4													# correct	# of opp.	%
Opportunities or Session #	1	4	7	9															
Task accuracy	-	-	-	+															

Figure 5.8 Example data collected for task accuracy using the opportunity-based format of the Additional Behaviors Data Sheet.

Scoring: (+) correct; (–) incorrect; On-task (+) scored if no more than 2 (minutes)/seconds off task

Date	6/1	6/1	6/4																# correct	# of opp.	%
Opportunities or Session #	1	4	7	9																	
On-task	–	+	+	–																	

Figure 5.9 Example data collected for on-task behavior using the opportunity-based format of the Additional Behaviors Data Sheet.

assigned task. The criteria is indicated in the top portion of the data sheet, as shown in Figure 5.9.

As illustrated in Figure 5.9, the data collector records the session number in each box of the second row. Note that the data collector only includes sessions with the pre-specified opportunity to score this behavior, as indicated in the definition of on-task behavior earlier in the chapter (i.e., assignment of a particular task that is within the learner's repertoire, and the learner is given clear instructions and all necessary materials). Below this row, the data collector scores a "+" or a "–" in each box to indicate whether or not the learner remained on-task while working on the corresponding assigned task. It is recommended to document the criteria for scoring a learner as on-task, as shown in Figure 5.9.

Using the *frequency-based format* of the **Additional Behaviors Data Sheet** to collect data is illustrated in Figure 5.10. In this example, the instructor is collecting data on the target of greeting others. This data sheet provides a way to document each occurrence of a behavior and, if desired, link them to specific work sessions or observation periods. As illustrated in Figure 5.10, the data collector enters the date, session number, and duration of the observation period in the first row of the data sheet. In the second row, the data collector places hash marks on the sheet each time the behavior occurs during the designated observation period. As discussed further in Chapter 6, it is often important to indicate the total duration of the observation period, as shown in Figure 5.10 next to the session number.

Using the **interval-based format** of the **Additional Behaviors Data Sheet** to collect data is illustrated in Figure 5.11. In this example, the instructor has chosen the interval-based format rather than the opportunity-based format to collect data on on-task behavior (described previously). This format might be selected when it is desirable to get more precise information about the learner's level of on-task behavior while working on assigned tasks. However, it is still easier than collecting data on the learner's behavior continuously throughout the assessment. As illustrated in Figure 5.11, the work session number from the VSSA plan, which indicates the particular assigned task, can be documented in the top left portion of the sheet next to the date. The next row in the left portion of the sheet includes a space to note the length of each interval (e.g., 5 minutes). The remaining adjacent boxes in this row show interval numbers to help the data collector keep track of the intervals. Below this row, the data collector scores a "Y" or a "N" in each box to indicate whether or not the learner was on task at the end of the interval. The number of boxes needed for a particular task will depend on the duration of the task and the interval length.

As noted previously, instructors can use these data collection systems to track a variety of other social and job-related behaviors. The following is a

Date/Session #/Time (min)	7/2 #1 7 min	7/2 #4 18 min	7/5 #5 2 min		Total #	Total min	Rate (#/min)
Greeting others	/ / / /	/ / / / / / / / / / / /					
Rate (#/min):							

Figure 5.10 Example data collected for greeting others using the frequency-based format of the Additional Behaviors Data Sheet.

Scoring: (Y) if the behavior occurred; (N) if the behavior did not occur

Session # __3__   Date __6/7__

(Interval Length: 5 min)	1	2	3	4	5	6	7	8	9	10	11	12	13	14	15	16	17	18	19	20	# Yes	# of intervals	%
On-task	Y	Y	Y	N	Y	N	N	N	N														

Figure 5.11 Example data collected for on-task behaviors using the interval-based format of the Additional Behaviors Data Sheet.

list of some additional, potential responses with the recommended data collection formats in parentheses.

- Greeting others (frequency-based)
- Complimenting others (frequency-based)
- Thanking others (opportunity-based)
- Responding to safety hazards (opportunity-based)
- Standing an appropriate distance from others (opportunity- or interval-based)
- Waiting turn to speak (opportunity based)
- Asking appropriate questions (frequency-based)

Prior to data collection, the instructor will need to establish clear and objective definitions of any additional social and job-related behaviors that they want to track during the assessment. A summary of guidelines for defining behaviors, as discussed previously in this chapter, can be found in Appendix A.

In addition to these appropriate behaviors, it may be important to document occurrences of inappropriate behavior during the VSSA. Recommended systems for doing so are described in the next section.

Inappropriate Behavior

Inappropriate behavior, which can range from engaging in conversation that is inappropriate for the workplace (e.g., asking personal questions) to physical aggression, also can be important to document during the assessment. The frequency-based or interval-based formats of the **Additional Behaviors Data Sheet**, described previously, may be useful for gathering baseline (pre-intervention) data on levels of inappropriate behavior. A second data collection form, the **Functional Behavior Assessment Data Sheet,** is designed to obtain information that can be useful for identifying potential functions or reasons that the behavior occurs. This form can be found in Appendix B. Instructors can use this data sheet to document the situations that tend to proceed occurrences of the target (i.e., antecedents) and the events that immediately follow it (i.e., consequences). As discussed in Chapter 6, information about the function can help the instructor identify and teach relevant replacement behaviors (see also the case examples in Chapters 7 and 12).

As noted previously, the instructor should establish clear and objective definitions of the inappropriate behaviors that they want to track during the assessment. Asking caregivers and others who are familiar with the learner to describe the inappropriate behavior can be very helpful. Ideally, the instructor should create the definitions after observing the behaviors first-hand. The definitions should be as clear and complete as possible.

The definition also should include only observable characteristics. The following are some examples:

- Aggression: Hitting, kicking, or pushing others
- Yelling: Speaking above conversation level
- Property Destruction: Throwing, tearing, or breaking objects
- Elopement: Leaving or attempting to leave the workplace without permission

A summary of guidelines for defining behaviors, as discussed previously is this chapter, can be found in Appendix A.

Example data collected on inappropriate behavior using the ***interval-based format*** of the ***Additional Behaviors Data Sheet*** is illustrated in Figure 5.12. This format might be selected when the learner engages in high frequencies of the selected inappropriate responses and ease of recording is a priority over gaining more precise information about responding. As noted previously, interval lengths that do not exceed 5 minutes can provide a reasonably good estimate of the overall level of responding. This data sheet permits the data collector to record the occurrence (Y) or non-occurrence (N) of up to three different behaviors in each interval. The name of each behavior is entered in the left column of this sheet.

Example data collected on inappropriate behavior using the ***frequency-based format*** of the ***Additional Behaviors Data Sheet*** is illustrated in Figure 5.13. This option is useful when it is desirable to get more precise information about the learner's level of inappropriate behavior, and the behavior does not occur at frequencies that would make it difficult to record each occurrence. In the top row, the data collector records the date, the session number from the VSSA plan to link the data to the arranged situations and assigned tasks of the VSSA, and the duration of each session. Below this row, the data collector can record occurrences of different behaviors in each observation period. The name of each behavior is entered in the left column of this sheet. The data collector records a hashmark in one or more of the rows to document each time the learner engages in the behavior listed in the corresponding row.

As noted previously, it is often beneficial to use the ***Functional Behavior Assessment Data Sheet*** to obtain information about the antecedents and consequences of inappropriate behavior. As illustrated in Figure 5.14, the data sheet features an antecedent, behavior, and consequence (ABC) section to document situations that might be causing the inappropriate behavior. This section is pre-filled with antecedents and consequences that may occur during the VSSA, along with some blank spaces for the data collector to record other antecedents and consequences that arise. Definitions for the pre-filled events are provided in Table 5.2.

Scoring: (Y) if the behavior occurred; (N) if the behavior did not occur

Session # ___8___   Date ___6/10___

(Interval Length: 5 min.)	1	2	3	4	5	6	7	8	9	10	11	12	13	14	15	16	17	18	19	20	# Yes	# of intervals	%
Inappropriate statement	Y	Y	Y	Y	Y	N	Y	Y	Y	N	N	N											
Aggression	N	N	N	N	Y	N	N	N	N	N	N	N											
Wandering from work station	N	N	N	N	N	N	N	N	N	N	Y	Y											

Figure 5.12 Example data collected on inappropriate behavior using the interval-based format of the Additional Behaviors Data Sheet.

Date/Session #/Time (min)	6/1 #2 10min	6/2 #6 10min	6/5 #7 5min		Total #	Total min	Rate (#/min)
Aggression		/					
Rate (#/min):							
Yelling	/	////	//				
Rate (#/min):							

Figure 5.13 Example data collected on inappropriate behavior using the frequency-based format of the Additional Behaviors Data Sheet.

Learner: ____John_____	**Functional Behavior Assessment**	Instructor: __DL_____
Date: ___6/1/22___	**Data Sheet**	Data Collector: ___CW____

Target Behavior:	Definition:
Aggression	Hitting, kicking, punching others

Immediate Antecedent	Scoring: (X) for each instance of the behavior											Attention	Escape	Tangible
												Total # of Instances		
Supervisor unavailable														
Ignored by others														
Provided feedback	X													
Task interrupted			X											
Coworker asks for assistance			X											
Given clear instruction		X	X											
Given vague instruction														
Task not in repertoire														
Materials needed				X										
Conversing with peer														
Denied access to items/activities				X										

Immediate consequence

Given feedback/attention	X													
Ignored		X	X											
Task delayed or removed	X													
Provided items/activities				X										
Provided break		X												
Totals:														

If the highest number of instances of the target behavior were scored as **attention**, this indicates the learner most likely engages in the target behavior to access attention; this may be in the form of conversation, reprimands, or a reaction.

If the highest number of instances of the target behavior were scored as **escape**, this indicates the learner most likely engages in the target behavior to avoid work, get out of completing certain tasks, or get a break.

If the highest number of instances of the target behavior were scored as **tangible**, this indicates the learner most likely engages in the target behavior to gain access to an item or activity such as food, electronics, or personal items.

Figure 5.14 Example antecedent and consequence data collected on hitting, kicking, and punching using the Functional Behavior Assessment Data Sheet.

In the example in Figure 5.14, the participant was reported to engage in physical aggression, which is listed and defined at the top of the sheet. Each time the learner emits this behavior, the data collector notes what happened immediately before the aggression (the antecedent), and what happened immediately after the aggression (the consequence) by placing "X" marks in the corresponding boxes in each column. As shown in this example, the data collector selects multiple antecedents and consequences

Table 5.2 Definitions for the pre-filled events listed on the Functional Assessment Data Sheet.

Immediate Antecedent (event occurs just prior to behavior)	Example Definitions of Antecedents
Supervisor unavailable	Supervisor is with another person, on the phone, not in their expected location, or otherwise preoccupied when learner seeks assistance.
Ignored by others	Learner requests attention or initiates an interaction with someone who does not respond or reciprocate the interaction.
Provided feedback	Learner is given corrective feedback on performance (e.g, "Do a more thorough job", "move more quickly", "this is incorrect; do it this way instead".
Task Interrupted	Learner is asked to switch to a different task before completing the current assignment.
Coworker asks for assistance	A coworker requests help from the learner.
Given clear instructions	Learner is provided with all instructions and a demonstration when assigned a task.
Given vague instructions	The learner is provided incomplete and/or nonspecific instructions to complete a task that may be completed in different ways.
Task not in repertoire	The learner is assigned a task that is outside of their skill set or that includes a component for which they do not have the prerequisite skills.
Materials needed	The learner cannot complete their assigned task because the necessary materials are missing, broken, or of insufficient quantity.
Conversing with peer	Learner is interacting with a peer.
Denied access to items/activities	Learner has requested or attempted to access items but was told, "no," "wait until later," or was physically prevented access to the item or activity in some way.

Immediate Consequence (event occurs just after the behavior)	Example Definitions of Consequences
Given feedback/attention	Supervisor, staff, or a peer reacts to behavior with statements of concern, reprimands ("that's not nice, don't do that"), attempts to redirect verbally, or by talking about the learner's behavior to others within earshot.
Ignore	Nothing in the environment changes, and no one provides vocal or physical contact with the learner.
Task delayed/removed	Learner does not immediately return to an ongoing task following the behavior, or someone removes the work materials
Provided activity/items	Learner accesses an item or activity or someone gives them access to an item or activity.
Provided break	Supervisor or staff provide a formal break from work and permits the learner to go cool off or collect themselves.

when more than one occurs for a given instance of aggression. For example, the data collector has selected "provided feedback" as the antecedent and "given feedback/attention" and "task delayed or removed" as the consequences for the first instance of the behavior in Figure 5.14. At the conclusion of the assessment, these data are examined to develop hypotheses about the functions of behavior and how best to address these functions as part of the intervention. Chapter 6 provides more details about how to summarize and evaluate the data collected on the **Functional Behavior Assessment Data Sheet.**

Case Example

Let's now return to the case example of John from Chapter 4. His instructor, Charise, had decided to include all of the situations on the pre-filled Arranged Situations Data Sheet in Appendix B, along with some additional situations listed in the VSSA protocols that she felt might be most relevant to his likely job placements (instructed to relay information, provided multiple tasks, and prompted to take a designated break). Finally, based on information provided by John's teacher, Charise decided to include a time-pressure situation and selected targeted appropriate responses for this situation. To prepare her VSSA data collection system, she uses the template version of the **Arranged Situations Data Sheet** to include all of these situations.

Charise's next step was to consider other behaviors that might be useful to measure during John's VSSA. From the list of additional behaviors described in this chapter, Charise selected (a) confirming statements, (b) on-task behavior, and (c) inappropriate behavior. She excluded eye contact/orientation because she noticed that he gave good eye contact throughout the initial interview, which she plans to note in her final report to John's vocational counselor. She decided to document John's confirming statements because she felt that he might build better rapport with his supervisors by emitting confirming statements at least occasionally in response to task instructions. She decided to measure on-task behavior and inappropriate behavior because his teachers and parents identified potential problems when John was given nonpreferred tasks or told to complete tasks in a short period of time.

Charise's next step was to decide how she would collect data on these additional behaviors. After considering the three options for on-task behavior provided on the **Additional Behaviors Data Sheets** in the VSSA protocols, Charise selected the **opportunity-based** measurement system because John's teacher and parents reported that he generally remained on task, with some exceptions; thus, a less precise measurement system likely would be adequate. For this option, Charise needed to establish a criterion for scoring John as "on task" during each assigned task and decided that he would be considered on task as long as he did not stop working for more than one minute (excluding bathroom trips).

After considering the options for scoring inappropriate behavior provided on the ***Additional Behaviors Data Sheets***, Charise chose the ***frequency-based*** data collection system. She anticipated that he would engage in low occurrences of these behaviors, so they would be easy to track and link to specific assigned tasks throughout the assessment. For the specific inappropriate behaviors to document, Charise tentatively planned to collect data on task refusal statements and yelling, as reported by John's teacher and parents during the interview. To successfully track inappropriate behavior, Charise must establish clear definitions of the behaviors. Using the guidelines provided in this chapter, Charise drafted the following definitions based on the descriptions provided by John's teacher and parents:

- Behavior #1: Task Refusal – John's task refusals occur when he makes statements indicating that he will not follow a direction or complete a task (e.g., saying, "no" or "I don't want to do that.") even if he complies. Data should only be collected when someone has given him an instruction or assigned him a task. Task refusals do not include statements about optional activities or when rejecting a choice.
- Behavior #2: Yelling- John's yelling occurs when he vocalizes above conversation level. Yelling does not include laughing or attempts to get someone's attention from a distance.

Charise also considered the possibility of collecting data using the ***Functional Behavior Assessment Data Sheet*** to obtain information about the antecedents and consequences of inappropriate behavior. However, she decided to wait until she obtained some of the initial results of the assessment. If levels of inappropriate behavior indicated that it would be a primary concern, Charise would be prepared to gather information about the common antecedents and consequences of the behavior. The results of John's assessment, along with a description of how Charise summarized, analyzed, and interpreted these data, are presented in Chapter 6.

6 Summarizing and Interpreting VSSA Results

A completed VSSA permits the instructor to (a) identify the learner's strengths and areas for improvement, (b) share assessment findings with the learner and other stakeholders, and (c) prioritize targets for intervention. Accomplishing these goals requires a number of steps. First, the instructor will need to summarize the data collected during the VSSA. Second, the instructor will need to analyze and interpret the results, a process that is greatly eased by graphing the data or using the reporting forms provided in Appendix B. Third, the instructor will need to create easy-to-understand reports and displays to share with the learner and stakeholders. Finally, in collaboration with the learner and stakeholders, the instructor will need to prioritize the targets for intervention. This chapter provides detailed instructions and examples for completing these steps and concludes with the case example (John) presented in the prior chapters.

Summarizing the Data

After completing the VSSA, the instructor likely will have multiple data sheets, each containing a variety of scores and information about the learner's performance. The first step in summarizing the data is to collapse the information collected across multiple observations and situations. This information is then transferred to the *VSSA Results Report Form*, which can replace more traditional graphs. The following sections describe how to summarize and report data from the VSSA.

Arranged Situations Data Sheet

Each section in the *Arranged Situations Data Sheet* contains an area for summarizing the data collected for that particular arranged situation. This area appears at the end of each row assigned to each targeted behavior for that situation. If the instructor used multiple data sheets to record data on the learner's response(s) when encountering the arranged situation, the simplest approach is to use the summary section on just one

DOI: 10.4324/9781003311935-6

Vague Instructions/Task not in Repertoire

Session #	4	5	10	14	20		# correct	# of opp.	%
Seeks assistance	-	+	+	+	+		4	5	80%
Makes help statement	+	+	+	+	+		5	5	100%

Figure 6.1 Example of summarized data on the Arranged Situations Data Sheet.

sheet (e.g., the final one) to summarize all of the data on that response collected during the VSSA.

It is recommended to summarize these data by determining the percentage of opportunities with a correct response for each targeted learner behavior. To complete this calculation, the instructor uses the designated summary boxes at the end of each row, as illustrated in Figure 6.1. The instructor totals the number of correct responses ("+") and enters this sum in the first box (under "# correct"). The instructor then determines the total number of times the learner had an opportunity to perform the response by summing the correct ("+") and incorrect ("–") responses ("+" plus "–") and entering this sum in the second box (under "# of opp."). The instructor then calculates the percentage by dividing the number of correct responses by the total number of opportunities and converting it to a percentage (i.e., multiply by 100). As illustrated in Figure 6.1, this percentage is listed in the last box (under "%").

Additional Behaviors Data Sheet

Similar to the Arranged Situations Data Sheet, the **Additional Behaviors Data Sheets** include areas for summarizing the data collected on each behavior. These areas appear at the end of each row. If the instructor used multiple data sheets to record data on the learner's response during the VSSA, it is recommended to use the summary section on just one sheet (e.g., the final one) to summarize all of the data. The method used to summarize the data depends on the particular measurement system used.

Opportunity-based Recording

As described in Chapter 5, the instructor will score a response as correct ("+") or incorrect ("–") during each opportunity when using this recording format. It is recommended to determine the percentage of opportunities with a correct response for each targeted response. Similar to the calculations for behaviors on the Arranged Situations Data Sheet, the instructor uses the designated summary boxes at the end of each row to record the total number of correct responses ("+") and the total

Scoring: (+) correct; (−) incorrect; On-task (+) scored if no more than 5 minutes / seconds off task

Date	8/1	8/1	8/1	8/3	8/3	8/5	8/5	8/5	8/8	# correct	# of opp.	%
Opportunities or Session #	1	3	4	6	8	11	12	14	15			
On-task	−	+	+	−	+	+	+	−	−	5	9	56%

Figure 6.2 Example of summarized data using the opportunity-based format of the Additional Behaviors Data Sheet.

number of times the learner had an opportunity to perform the response ("+" plus "−"). The instructor then determines the percentage by dividing the number of correct responses by the total number of opportunities converting it to a percentage (i.e., multiply by 100), as illustrated in Figure 6.2.

An important caveat should be noted. In Chapter 5, it was recommended that the instructor record the work session number, when relevant, in the box above the data collected on the behavior. This allows the instructor to link correct and incorrect responses to certain tasks or situations. However, the example summary just described collapses the data collected on behavior across all work and observation sessions. If a learner engages in higher or lower levels of behavior (e.g., on-task behavior or inappropriate behavior) when assigned certain tasks, this data summary would obscure this important outcome. For this reason, the instructor should closely inspect the data sheets for such patterns during the summary process.

Interval-based Recording

Similar to the opportunity-based format, the instructor should sum the total number of intervals with a "Y" *across all observations* and divide this sum by the total number of observation intervals included in the VSSA. The product is then multiplied by 100 to convert it to a percentage. The total number of observation intervals is determined by summing the total "Y" and "N" as illustrated in Figure 6.3.

Scoring: (Y) if the behavior occurred; (N) if the behavior did not occur

Session # ___3___ Date ___6/7_____

(Interval Length:_5 min_)	1	2	3	4	5	6	7	8	9	# Yes	# of intervals	%
On-task	Y	Y	Y	N	Y	N	N	N	N	4	9	44%

Figure 6.3 Example of summarized data using the interval-based format of the Additional Behaviors Data Sheet.

Frequency-based Recording

The data sheet for frequency-based recording provides three different ways to summarize the data, as illustrated in Figure 6.4. First, the instructor can sum the number of occurrences (hash marks) across all sessions or observations for each response and enter the number in the first box at the end of each row (under "Total #"). This provides an overall level of behavior that occurred during the VSSA for each response.

The instructor also can convert the frequency data to a rate (e.g., responses per minute). The data sheet permits the instructor to calculate the rate in two different ways. First, the instructor can sum the total number of minutes across all sessions or observations for each response, enter the number in the second box at the end of each row (under "Total min"), divide the total number of occurrences by the total time, and then enter this outcome in the last box of each row (under "Rate[#/min]). Second, the instructor can convert the frequency data to a rate for each session or observation by dividing the number of hash marks in each column by the total minutes of the observation and entering this outcome in the last row of each column (next to "Rate [#/min]").

Calculating rate is desirable when comparing levels of responding across varied observation lengths. Further, the instructor might calculate the rate when (a) comparing levels of behavior across specific assigned tasks or situations, (b) comparing levels of different behaviors, or (c) evaluating levels of behavior across repeated sessions or observations, as discussed for the VSSI in Chapter 10. The data in Figure 6.4 illustrate one advantage of calculating rate when summarizing and interpreting results from the VSSA. Notice that the learner engaged in 2 instances of self-injury during Session #4 (first data column) and 10 instances of self-injury during Session #12 (second data column). Suppose the instructor looks at the VSSA plan and notices that they had asked the learner to complete a shirt-folding task in Session #4 and a vacuuming task in Session #12. A comparison of the overall frequency of self-injury associated with each task suggests that the learner engaged in much more self-injury when vacuuming than when folding shirts (10 instances versus 2 instances). The instructor might speculate that vacuuming was more aversive to the learner. However, as indicated inthe top row of the data sheet, Session #4 lasted just 5 minutes whereas Session # 12 lasted 20 minutes. Converting the frequency data to a

Date/Session #/Time (min)	6/1 #4 5 min	6/2 #12 20 min	Total #	Total min	Rate (#/min)
Self-injury	//	//////////	12	25	0.48
Rate (#/min):	0.4	0.5			

Figure 6.4 Example of summarized data using the frequency-based format of the Additional Behaviors Data Sheet.

rate, which takes the observation time into account, suggests that the learner engaged in similar levels of inappropriate behavior when assigned those tasks (0.4 responses per minute for folding and 0.5 for vacuuming; see bottom row of Figure 6.4).

This example also raises the important caveat noted earlier in the chapter about the potential to obscure important differences in responding across tasks or situations if the data are collapsed across all observations. Thus, when using frequency-based data collection, it is recommended that the instructor closely inspect the data sheets for such patterns during the summary process.

Functional Behavior Assessment Data Sheet

Like the other sheets, the **Functional Behavior Assessment Data Sheet** includes guidance on how best to summarize the data collected during the VSSA. In this case, however, the focus of the summary is on the antecedents and consequences that are checked during the assessment. The areas at the end of each row in the antecedents and consequences sections include boxes to record the total number of times that particular event was checked, as illustrated in Figure 6.5.

To guide the interpretation of the results, the instructor first fills in the designated boxes at the end of each row under the columns with the headings "attention," "escape," and "tangibles." These are three common functions of inappropriate behavior. The total number of times each event was checked is recorded in the designated boxes, which correspond to the most relevant function or functions for that particular event. The instructor should enter the same number in all boxes that appear in the same row. Boxes with light grey borders appear at the end of the blank rows that the instructor might use to record antecedents and consequences that do not appear in the pre-filled data sheet. These boxes indicate that the instructor will need to make an educated guess about the most relevant function(s) associated with any documented events. Suppose, for example, that the instructor recorded the presence of loud noises as an antecedent to inappropriate behavior. The instructor might speculate that an escape function (escape from aversive noise) is most relevant to this antecedent. If so, the instructor would enter the number of times that this occurred in the box under the escape column.

After completing the boxes, the instructor then sums the numbers in each column and enters the total number in the bottom row to obtain information about the potential function(s) of the inappropriate behavior. Relatively high totals for specific function(s) provides evidence to support hypotheses regarding those functions. For example, based on the data shown in Figure 6.5 the instructor might hypothesize that the learner's inappropriate behavior is maintained by escape from aversive events.

Immediate Antecedent	Scoring: (X) for each instance of the behavior	Attention	Escape	Tangible
		Total # of Instances		
Supervisor unavailable		0		
Ignored by others		0		
Provided feedback	X		1	
Task interrupted	X		1	
Coworker asks for assistance	X		1	
Given clear instruction	X X		2	
Given vague instruction			0	
Given task not in repertoire			0	
Materials needed	X			1
Conversing with peer		0	0	0
Denied access to items/activities	X			1

Immediate consequence	Scoring	Attention	Escape	Tangible
Given feedback/attention		0		
Ignored	X X X		3	
Task delayed or removed			0	
Provided items/activities	X			1
Provided break	X X		2	2
Totals:		0	10	5

If the highest number of instances of the target behavior were scored as **attention**, this indicates the learner most likely engages in the target behavior to access attention; this may be in the form of conversation, reprimands, or a reaction.

If the highest number of instances of the target behavior were scored as **escape**, this indicates the learner most likely engages in the target behavior to avoid work, get out of completing certain tasks, or get a break.

If the highest number of instances of the target behavior were scored as **tangible**, this indicates the learner most likely engages in the target behavior to gain access to an item or activity such as food, electronics, or personal items.

Figure 6.5 Example data summary on the Functional Behavior Assessment Data Sheet.

Compiling and Reporting the Results

Once the instructor summarizes all of the data, the summaries may be easily transferred to the *VSSA Results Report Form* provided in Appendix B. This sheet enables the instructor to compile all results in a manner that is easy to review and share with others. Moreover, the sheet provides a visual display that facilitates data interpretation and selection of targets for instruction that is typically afforded by traditional graphic data displays. As such, the *VSSA Results Report Form* can eliminate the need for graphing.

Appendix B includes two variations of this form, one labeled "Sample" and the other labeled "Template." The Sample is pre-filled with the "standard" (i.e., recommended) situations and associated responses that might be included in the VSSA. The template version contains no pre-filled situations or responses. The instructor would use this version if they arranged situations or collected data on responses that are not included on the sample data sheet or in the VSSA protocol.

The "Sample" version has separate spaces to record the summary data for each response that could have occurred during the situation (if more than one), as illustrated in Figure 6.6. These responses are listed at the

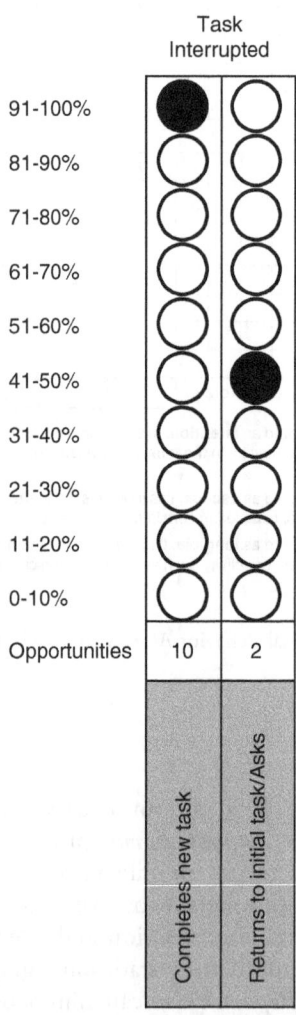

Figure 6.6 Example results on the VSSA Results Report Form.

bottom of each section. A row of unfilled circles appears in the column above each response, with each circle corresponding to a range of percentages (e.g., 91% to 100%), which are listed to the left of each section. The instructor simply fills in the circle that aligns with the range that includes the percentage obtained for that learner. For example, if the learner engaged in a response during 95% of opportunities, the instructor would select the circle that aligns with the range 91%–100%, as illustrated in Figure 6.6.

The row immediately above the listed responses in each section contains boxes to record the total number of opportunities that the learner had to engage in the response during the VSSA. This information might enhance understanding of the results, particularly if the learner had very few opportunities to perform the response. For example, suppose the instructor reports that the learner exhibited a correct response on 50% of the opportunities to do so, as shown in the second column in Figure 6.6. Knowing that the learner had just two opportunities to perform that response (versus, for example, 10 opportunities) might suggest that the VSSA did not capture an adequate sample of performance for that response. The "Template" version is identical to the "Sample," but requires the instructor to enter the situations and associated responses.

Tables to record the results for behaviors tracked on the ***Additional Behaviors Data Sheet***s appear below the sections for the arranged situations. As shown in Figure 6.7, separate tables are provided to summarize the data collected for additional appropriate and inappropriate behaviors. Up to eight different behaviors can be entered across the two tables. After listing each behavior in the boxes under the heading "behavior," the instructor would transfer the data summaries they completed as described in Chapter 5 by entering either a percentage (for opportunity-based and interval-based recording) or the total number or rate (for frequency-based recording) in the boxes under the heading "% / # / Rate."

Additional Behaviors

Behavior	% / # / Rate	Behavior	% / # / Rate

Inappropriate Behaviors

Behavior	% / # / Rate	Behavior	% / # / Rate

Figure 6.7 Tables to record results for additional appropriate and inappropriate behaviors on the VSSA Results Report Form.

As discussed earlier in this chapter, this summary collapses the data collected on behavior(s) across all work and observation sessions. This might obscure important differences in responding that are associated with different tasks or situations. If a close inspection of the data sheets reveals these potentially important patterns, the instructor could consider adding additional tables or comments to the report form to share this information.

If the instructor collected data on the antecedents and consequences of inappropriate behavior, the **Functional Behavior Assessment Data Sheet** can serve as a reporting form to convey information about the hypothesized function(s) of the behavior.

Interpreting and Sharing the Results

Once the instructor has summarized and displayed the results on the **VSSA Results Report Form** or through other graphic displays, the instructor is ready to share the results with the learner and other stakeholders (e.g., parents and teachers). This section describes how to inspect the data recorded on the **Results Report Form** to identify the learner's strengths, areas for improvement, and targets to prioritize for instruction.

The filled circles indicating performance for each response can be visually inspected to easily identify responses with high and low levels of performance. Level of performance corresponds directly to the placement of the filled circle in the column. Thus, the higher (or lower) the filled circle's placement in the column, the higher (or lower) the learner's level of performance during the VSSA. A quick scan of the Results Reporting Form can reveal a learner's strengths and potential areas for instruction and these findings are shared with the learner and stakeholders.

Decisions about whether to target responses associated with specific arranged situations or other behaviors tracked during the VSSA will depend on a variety of factors, including the learner's planned job placement(s), preferred job settings or tasks, and the priorities of the learner and stakeholders. The instructor, learner, and other stakeholders might consider the types of situations that the learner is likely to encounter on particular jobs and the typical practices or expectations of workers in those settings.

For example, suppose a learner desires a job assembling electronic parts for computers. Information obtained about this particular job placement indicates that employees rarely, if ever, encounter broken or missing materials and are expected to remain at their workstations. Thus, searching for needed materials is not particularly relevant to success on this job and may not be considered a priority target for this learner. Suppose that another learner has prioritized jobs that require a great deal of interaction with customers and coworkers. In this case, targets that may improve social relationships (e.g., offering assistance, making confirming statements, orienting towards others when speaking or listening) may be considered particularly important to target for this learner.

For learners who engaged in significant levels of inappropriate behavior during the VSSA, information obtained from the ***Functional Behavior Assessment Data Sheet*** may offer important additional considerations when selecting targets. As noted previously, the focus of these protocols is to build appropriate responses to replace inappropriate behaviors that occur during problematic situations rather than targeting the reduction of inappropriate behavior per se. Thus, identifying the conditions under which they occur and the possible reinforcing consequences that maintain these behaviors should help guide subsequent intervention. This information will be used in several different ways.

First, any identified problematic situations (i.e., antecedents) that are likely to occur on the current or planned job site should be arranged during the VSSI so that the learner can practice appropriate replacement behaviors within the context of those situations. Second, the instructor should target appropriate behaviors that likely will lead to the same reinforcers that maintain the inappropriate behavior. For example, suppose the hypothesized function of inappropriate behavior is escape from certain tasks. Targeted alternative replacement behaviors might include asking for a break from work or for help completing the task.

In some cases, the instructor may have difficulty identifying hypothesized functions despite careful documentation on the ***Functional Behavior Assessment Data Sheet***. This might occur when the instructor often does not notice any obvious antecedents or consequences to document on the data sheet or when the inappropriate behavior occurs infrequently during the assessment. It also might be difficult to use the data to guide intervention planning when the instructor documents numerous different antecedents and consequences on the data sheet, resulting in multiple hypothesized functions. In such cases, identifying and reinforcing the types of appropriate social- and problem-solving behaviors recommended in this book is still the best course of action. To do so, the instructor will need to identify and deliver potent reinforcers for these behaviors using the strategies discussed in Chapters 3 and 9. The desired outcome is for the learner to engage in these appropriate behaviors instead of the inappropriate ones.

Additional considerations for selecting targets for intervention will be discussed within the context of the case examples in the next section (John) and in Chapters 7 and 12.

Case Example

John's instructor, Charise, completed the VSSA using the plan and data collection system described in Chapters 4 and 5. Next, she summarized, evaluated, and shared the results with John, his parents, and his vocational rehabilitation counselor. Her first step, as described previously in this chapter, was to summarize the results obtained on her various data sheets across the assessment. She began with the ***Arranged Situations***

Data Sheet. An example of her calculations for one of the situations (supervisor unavailable) is shown in Figure 6.8, and a summary of all her calculations for John's responses during the VSSA is displayed in Table 6.1

Next, Charise summarized the responses that she tracked on the ***Additional Behavior Data Sheets.*** As described in Chapter 5, Charise collected data on confirming statements and on-task behavior using the opportunity-based format of the data sheet and on inappropriate behavior using the frequency-based format of the sheet. As Charise was summarizing the data collected for John's on-task behavior, shown in Figure 6.9, she noticed that he was only off-task during sessions with a time-pressure situation (i.e., when he was told to complete a task in a

Supervisor Unavailable

Session #	4	6	17			# correct	# of opp.	%
Returns to work area	+	+	+			3	3	100%
Begins additional task	-	-	-			0	3	0%

Scoring: (+) correct; (-) incorrect, (N) no opportunity

Figure 6.8 Summary of data collected during the supervisor-unavailable situation for John's VSSA.

Table 6.1 Summary of John's performance during the arranged situations of the VSSA; N/O = no opportunity because all feedback was clear

---

Arranged Situations, Responses, & Percentage of Opportunities With Correct Responses

---

Task Interrupted
• Completes new task = 100%
• Returns to initial task = 0%

Materials Needed
• Searches for materials = 60%
• Finds materials = 100%
• Seeks assistance = 100%
• Requests help = 100%
Vague-Instructions/Task-Not-in-Repertoire
• Seeks assistance = 50%
• Requests help = 50%
Feedback Provided
• Acknowledges feedback = 0%
• Asks for clear feedback = N/O
• Confirms understanding = 0%
• Corrects mistake = 100%
Time Pressure
• Seeks assistance = 0%
• Requests help = 0%

Task Completed
• Seeks supervisor = 100%
• Says "finished" = 100%
• Asks for next task = 78%
Supervisor Unavailable
• Returns to work area = 100%
• Begins additional task = 0%

Multiple Tasks
• Transitions = 100%

Relay Information
• Delivers information = 100%

End of Break
• Resumes work = 100%

Scoring: (+) correct; (−) incorrect; On-task (+) scored if no more than _1_ minute off task

Date	3/15	3/15	3/15	3/15	3/15	3/15	3/15	3/16	3/16	3/16	3/16	3/16	3/16	# correct	# of opp.	%
Opportunities/Session #	1	2	3	4	7	9	10	11	12	14	16	18	19			
On-Task	+	−	+	+	+	−	+	+	+	+	+	−	+	10	13	77%

Figure 6.9 Summary of data collected on John's on-task behavior using the opportunity-based format of the Additional Behaviors Data Sheet.

limited amount of time). She identified this pattern by linking the session numbers listed on the sheet to the arranged situations in his VSSA plan. (Note that some sessions do not appear in Figure 6.9 because Charise only collected data on on-task behavior when he had clear instructions and all materials needed to complete the task.) These results tell Charise that the type of assigned task (i.e., preferred versus nonpreferred) did not seem relevant to his on-task behavior. Charise had noticed a similar pattern while collecting data on John's inappropriate behavior. In fact, John only exhibited inappropriate behavior during three tasks, and all occurred during a time-pressure situation. Because John rarely exhibited inappropriate behavior during the assessment and because Charise observed a predictable antecedent to his behavior (time pressure statement), she did not collect functional behavior assessment data during the VSSA.

After Charise summarized all of her data, she compiled the results by transferring them to the *VSSA Results Report Form* so that she could share the information with John, his vocational counselor, and his parents. As shown in Figure 6.10, she used the top portion of the template reporting form to display the results from the *Arranged Situations Data Collection Sheet* and the bottom portion of the form to display the summary data from the *Additional Behaviors Data Sheets*. (Note that only a portion of John's arranged situations data are shown in Figure 6.10, as the template form has space for up to seven situations, with any remaining data reported on a second page of the form.)

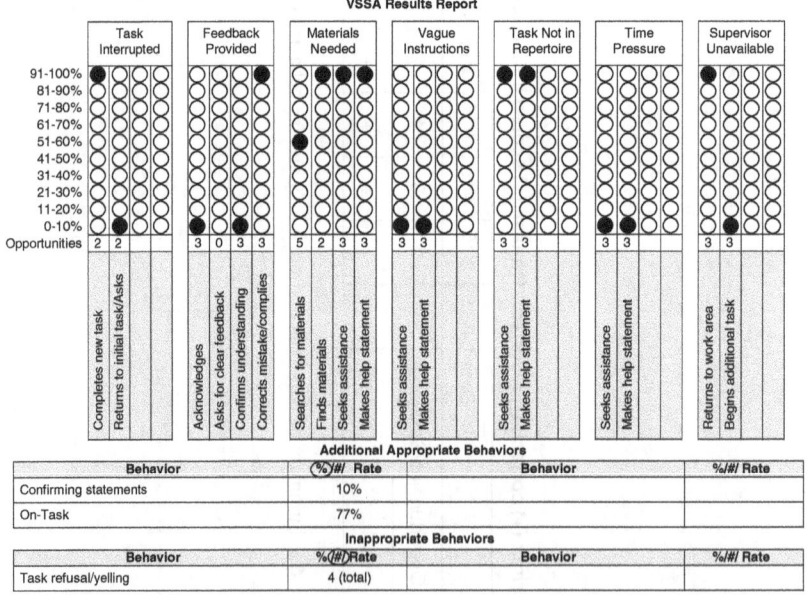

Figure 6.10 John's VSSA Results Report.

Next, Charise met with John, his vocational counselor, and his parents to review and discuss the results shown in Figure 6.10. Charise first emphasized John's numerous strengths, noting that he always switched to a newly assigned task when she interrupted his current task, requested help with broken or missing materials, asked for help when given a task that was clearly outside of his skill set, notified his supervisor when he completed his work, correctly relayed information to others, transitioned independently across multiple assigned tasks, and corrected his mistakes when Charise provided feedback. In addition, John always resumed his work as soon as his designated break times ended.

Charise then discussed several key skill areas that John might want to target for improvement. While doing so, she asked for the group's input on the skills and associated situations to prioritize for intervention. In their discussion, they considered John's job preferences and the relative importance of the different skills for helping John obtain and maintain employment. In particular, John found it difficult to manage time-pressure situations by remaining calm and asking for help. This was particularly concerning in light of John's desire to work in fast food or other busy retail businesses. Charise also noted that John often did not seek assistance or ask for help when he was given vague instructions and, thus, was not certain how to complete a task. John and his parents agreed that this was likely a skill he would need to be successful and particularly critical during the early stages of employment.

John's vocational counselor pointed to the data showing that John never looked for other work to complete when his supervisor was not available to assist him. As such, he remained unoccupied until his supervisor was free, which might reflect poorly on his job performance. Finally, among the remaining possible targets, Charise noted that John might develop better relationships with future employers if he increased the frequency of his confirming statements and acknowledged his supervisor's feedback. With these factors in mind, John and Charise prioritized the following skills and associated situations:

- Confirm understanding of new task instructions and supervisor feedback
- Acknowledge feedback from your supervisor
- Ask for help when given a task that you don't know how to do
- Ask for help when given a deadline that is too difficult to meet
- Find additional work to do when the supervisor is unavailable

Charise's next steps for developing and implementing interventions for these skills are described in Chapter 8.

7 VSSA Case Examples

This chapter provides additional case examples to help illustrate the assessment process across a variety of learners, settings, and service delivery models. The goal is to provide exemplars of the different ways the VSSA may be tailored to meet the needs and goals of individual learners. All of the case examples are based on actual learners with whom my students and I have worked, with some changes to protect the confidentiality and anonymity of the individuals as well as to illustrate particular nuances for instructive purposes. These case examples are presented again in Chapter 12 to illustrate the VSSI.

Case Example #1: Sergio

Sergio is a 16-year-old student with autism and moderate intellectual disabilities who receives special education services in a public high school. Sergio uses an augmentative communication device to make requests and to initiate and respond to greetings. He communicates using the symbol-based software application Proloquo2Go® installed on an iPad®, which he carries with him in a bag strapped around his shoulders.

Sergio is receiving work experience in the cafeteria and school store on his high school campus. Thus far, Sergio's vocational goals have targeted following directions and completing assigned vocational tasks without prompts (e.g., sweeping the cafeteria and stocking the school store). Sergio's teacher and his parents would like to prepare Sergio for his first part-time job in the community by expanding his goals to include relevant social-communication and problem-solving targets. His teacher, Trina, plans to conduct the VSSA within the context of his vocational training on campus.

Step 1: Gather Information

His teacher, Trina, begins the process by meeting with Sergio, his parents, and a former teacher to obtain information pertinent to the VSSA that she could not answer herself. Using the interview form in Appendix A to guide her information gathering, Trina obtains the following relevant information:

DOI: 10.4324/9781003311935-7

- When asked, Sergio could not indicate his preferred job placements. However, his parents believe that he would do well in a retail store or restaurant. He seems to enjoy cleaning and stocking shelves.
- Sergio seems to prefer to work on tasks alone. He does not typically initiate interactions with others.
- At home, Sergio sweeps and vacuums the floors, washes the dishes, sets the table for dinner, and takes out the trash.
- Sergio knows how to complete a number of basic tasks, such as folding shirts, sorting objects, stapling, shredding paper, filling salt and pepper shakers, sweeping and mopping, wiping tables, and rolling silverware. He does not know how to use a computer, count change, or tell time with either a digital or analog clock.
- Sergio reads on a 1st-grade level.
- While working in the cafeteria and school store, Sergio follows most directions, remains on task with very little prompting, and can complete his assigned tasks correctly. However, he does not transition independently across tasks. Sergio will typically wait for his teacher to instruct him to start the next task when he has completed the previous one. For example, once he has finished sweeping the floor, he typically stands idle until his teacher notices that he has finished sweeping and tells him that he can start mopping.
- At both home and school, Sergio occasionally engages in disruptive behavior (i.e., yelling, sitting on the floor with arms folded) when his schedule changes or when he is given a brand-new task. His parents and teachers typically tell him to sit down and take a break from the activities when this occurs. When they do, he calms down fairly quickly. In most cases, he eventually agrees to resume the activities or tasks.

Step 2: Select the Arranged Situations

Trina decides to include most of the recommended situations outlined in the VSSA protocol, as she and Sergio's parents would like to identify and target relevant social and problem-solving skills that will help prepare him for employment. Trina also considers whether to include additional situations based on her own observations of Sergio. She knows that Sergio sometimes has problematic behavior with changes in his routine or when given brand-new tasks. Several of the recommended situations seem relevant to this situation, including the task-interrupted situation and the task-not-in-repertoire situation. Conducting the VSSA within the context of his regular work activities also would necessarily create changes in his regular routine. However, to be certain that she captures the full range of situations that might be difficult for Sergio, Trina plans to occasionally ask him to do tasks that she has never assigned him before.

Because Sergio may engage in inappropriate behavior during the VSSA, Trina also must plan how she will react to this behavior. As recommended

Table 7.1 Sergio's arranged situations for the VSSA

Task Interrupted
Materials Needed
Vague Instructions
Task Not in Repertoire
Feedback Provided (Clear)
Task Completed
Supervisor Unavailable
Multiple Tasks

in Chapter 4, Trina will respond to Sergio's behavior in the same way that people in his life typically do. In this case, she knows that his teachers and parents usually ask him to calm down and take a brief break from ongoing activities.

Finally, Trina is concerned that Sergio is too dependent on prompts to transition from one task to the next. The task-completed situation would permit her to formally assess his performance when she doesn't immediately step in to assist him. However, she would also like to assess his ability to transition across tasks when she tells him to complete a short sequence of multiple tasks. To do so, she will include a multiple-task situation with a fixed order for the tasks (i.e., "fixed sequence") because many of the tasks in the cafeteria and store must be completed in a certain order (e.g., Sergio must sweep the floor before he mops it; he must open the boxes of merchandise before he can stock the shelves). She plans to use the quick reference table for the multiple-task situation provided in Appendix A. Her final list of arranged situations is displayed in Table 7.1.

Step 3: Select the Tasks

Because Trina plans to conduct the VSSA within the context of Sergio's work activities in the cafeteria and school store on his campus, the VSSA will include his regularly assigned tasks. His responsibilities in the school cafeteria include sweeping and mopping the floors, wiping down the tables and chairs, and taking the trash out to the dumpster. His responsibilities in the school store include opening boxes, sorting merchandise, and stocking shelves. These tasks are consistent with his skills and preferences.

Trina also needs to consider tasks that would be appropriate for the vague-instructions and task-not-in-repertoire situations, which require tasks that Sergio does not routinely complete at school. These new task situations also will be useful for evaluating whether Sergio engages in problematic behavior when given new tasks, which Trina and Sergio's parents have anecdotally noticed. Trina knows that Sergio cannot count change or complete any computer-related tasks. She also does not believe that he would know how to take inventory if she instructed him to do so.

Making spreadsheets in Excel on the school store's computer, taking inventory of their merchandise, and counting money in the store's cash register would be appropriate for the task-not-in-repertoire situation. For the vague-instructions situation, Trina decided that she would assign him new cleaning tasks in the cafeteria and school store but omit the details about exactly how she would like him to complete the new cleaning tasks. Trina's final list of tasks, along with the possible situations that she could arrange when assigning those tasks, appears in Table 7.2. Note that the VSSA protocol does not recommend interrupting any tasks that are assigned to the vague-instructions or task-not-in-repertoire situations. Because Trina believes that the tasks selected for the task-not-in-repertoire situation will be quite difficult for Sergio, she does not combine it with any other situation (e.g., feedback, task completed) and will move on to the next task even if he correctly asks for help. If he does ask for help, she will simply state, "Thanks for asking for help but let's just move on to the next task." Trina can arrange to provide feedback during any of the other tasks and can arrange to be unavailable for any situation requiring his assistance.

Table 7.2 Sergio's selected tasks for the VSSA

Tasks	Potential Arranged Situations*
Store	
Opening boxes	Task Interrupted, Task Completed
Sorting merchandise	Task Interrupted, Task Completed
Stocking shelves	Task Interrupted, Task Completed
Cleaning shelves	Vague Instructions, Materials Needed
Cleaning the cash register	Vague Instructions, Materials Needed
Cleaning the glass cases	Vague Instructions, Materials Needed
Counting money in cash register	Task Not In Repertoire
Taking inventory	Task Not In Repertoire
Creating a spreadsheet in Excel	Task Not In Repertoire
Cafeteria	
Sweeping the floor	Task Interrupted, Materials Needed, Task Completed
Mopping the floor	Task Interrupted, Materials Needed, Task Completed
Wiping the tables and chairs	Task Interrupted, Materials Needed, Task Completed
Taking trash to dumpster	Task Completed
Cleaning the trays	Vague Instructions
Cleaning the garbage cans	Vague Instructions

* NOTES: Feedback can be delivered during any of Sergio's tasks; Supervisor Unavailable can be arranged for any situation requiring supervisor assistance. The multiple-task situation will be arranged by assigning up to three tasks from the list at one time.

Step 4: Select the Task Amounts

Sergio works in the cafeteria or school store during one 60-minute class period each day, three days per week. Trina wants to obtain an adequate sample of Sergio's social-communication and problem-solving skills during these class periods and does not want to prolong the VSSA. Thus, she feels that efficiency is going to be very important. While completing the VSSA, she will prioritize arranging opportunities to observe these skills rather than ensuring that he completes all of his usual assigned tasks. Thus, for example, he may not end up mopping all of the floor areas, opening all of the boxes, and stocking all of the shelves that he normally completes during these class periods. For any new tasks (e.g., cleaning the trays), she will select amounts that she feels Sergio could complete in no more than 10 minutes.

Step 5: Arrange the Environment

Next, Trina considers Sergio's current work environment and whether it may be beneficial to alter aspects of it during the VSSA. In terms of the work locations, Sergio typically moves to different areas of the cafeteria and store, depending on his current assigned task. However, none of the locations have a designated supply area that Sergio can access because his teacher provides him with all the necessary materials and closely monitors his progress to ensure that he has everything he needs. Trina wants to observe how Sergio responds when he is missing something he needs to complete a task. Thus, she assembles a cart that will have all the necessary supplies and plans to show him the location of the cart prior to the start of each class period.

Trina next considers her location. She typically remains in close proximity to Sergio so that she can provide him with the necessary materials and prompt him to transition to his next task. She would like to observe his performance when she isn't providing so much assistance. Thus, she establishes a location in the cafeteria and school store where she can remain some distance from Sergio but still observe him. She plans to sit at a table or desk and pretend to be busy working on something else. At the start of each new task, she will point out her planned location and remind him to let her know if he needs anything. During the supervisor-unavailable situation, she plans to pretend to have a conversation on her cell phone and will ignore any attempts to gain her attention at that time.

Finally, Trina considers Sergio's communication device, the iPad®, which he must use to interact with Trina during the VSSA. Although he typically carries it with him as he transitions across classes and activities throughout the day, Trina has noticed that Sergio does not always bring it with him when he works in the cafeteria or store. Instead, Sergio often leaves it in his homeroom. Because the goal of the VSSA is to assess social-communication skills, Trina will remind Sergio to always bring his

Table 7.3 Sergio's communication responses

Situation	Communication Response
Task Interrupted	N/A
Materials Needed	"Help"
Vague Instructions	"Help"
Task Not in Repertoire	"Help"
Feedback Provided (Clear)	"OK"
Task Completed	"Finished"
Supervisor Unavailable	N/A
Multiple Tasks	N/A

iPad®. She also will solicit assistance from his homeroom teacher to help ensure that he remembers to do so.

It is also important that communication responses relevant to the job site are available to Sergio when he launches the symbol-based software application. For example, he will need options to request assistance with materials or task instructions, or to inform his supervisor that he has completed a task. Trina knows that he has a generic "help" icon, which would be adequate for requesting assistance with materials or task instructions. Sergio has not yet learned how to request more precise help for job-related problems (e.g., requesting particular task materials) so Trina does not want to require this for the VSSA. He also has a "finished" icon that would be appropriate when notifying his supervisor of task completion and icons for communicating "OK" and "Yes" when acknowledging feedback and other instructions. Table 7.3 displays the communication responses that she selects for the relevant arranged situations.

Trina considers other possible responses to measure during the VSSA when she sets up her data collection plan, as discussed later in Step 7.

Step 6: Create the Assessment Plan

Next, Trina creates the assessment plan in Table 7.4 to help her stay organized and to ensure that she includes at least three opportunities for Sergio to experience each situation. She plans to arrange two multiple-task situations at the end of the assessment.

Step 7: Establish the Data Collection System

Once Trina has created her assessment plan, her next step is to determine how she will collect data on Sergio's performance during the VSSA. Trina plans to include all of the situations included on the ***Arranged Situations Sample Data Sheet*** discussed in Chapter 5 and provided in Appendix B, along with a multiple-tasks situation. In addition, she will modify some

Table 7.4 Sergio's Assessment Plan

Session	Task(s)	Arranged Situation(s)	Materials Needed
Sergio's Assessment Plan			
Cafeteria			
1	Sweep area	Materials Needed (dustpan on cart) Task Completed	Broom (dustpan missing)
2	Mop area (interrupt); Take trash to dumpster	Task Interrupted; Task Completed	Mop, soap, bucket
3	Clean 2 Trays	Vague Instructions; Clear Feedback; Task Completed	2 trays, soap, sponge, towels
Store			
4	Open 5 boxes	Task Completed; Supervisor Unavailable	5 boxes
5	Create Excel® spreadsheet	Task Not In Repertoire	Computer; data
6	Sort merchandise (interrupt); Clean 2 shelves	Task Interrupted; Task Completed	5 boxes; Sponge, paper towel roll
7	Count money	Task Not In Repertoire	Cash register, $1, $5, coins
Cafeteria			
8	Wipe 3 tables (interrupt) Take trash to dumpster	Task Interrupted; Task Completed; Supervisor Unavailable	Sponge, trash can
9	Clean 2 garbage cans	Vague Instructions; Clear Feedback; Task Completed	Lysol, paper towel roll
10	Wipe 20 chairs	Materials Needed (Wipes with supervisor); Supervisor Unavailable; Task Completed	Disinfecting wipes (remove all but one wipe)
Store			
11	Clean glass case	Vague Instructions Materials Needed (cloth with supervisor); Clear Feedback	Spray bottle (cloth missing)
12	Take inventory	Task Not In Repertoire	Paper, pencil
Cafeteria/Store			
13	Sweep area Mop area Trash to dumpster	Multiple Tasks	Broom, dustpan, mop, soap, bucket
14	Open boxes Sort merchandise Stock shelves	Multiple Tasks	5 boxes

of the definitions of correct responses printed on the sample sheet in light of the communication responses available on Sergio's device. As such, Trina will use the ***Arranged Situations Template Data Sheet*** provided in Appendix B so that she can include these modifications. An example of Trina's modifications to two of the arranged situations (vague

Vague Instructions/Task Not In Repertoire

Session #							# correct	# of opp.	%
Seeks assistance									
Presses "Help" icon									

Feedback Provided

Session #							# correct	# of opp.	%
Clear (C); Conflicting (F); Vague (V)									
Presses "OK" icon									
Corrects mistake									

Scoring: (+) correct; (-) incorrect, (N) no opportunity

Figure 7.1 Trina's modifications to the Arranged Situations Data Sheet for two situations included in Sergio's VSSA.

instructions/task not in repertoire and feedback provided) is shown in Figure 7.1.

Next, Trina considers other behaviors that she might want to measure by examining the potential additional behaviors mentioned in the protocol. Of these, Trina decides that confirming statements would be most appropriate for Sergio, given his current communication repertoire. For confirming statements, Trina will track whether Sergio activates the "OK" icon when given a new task instruction using the *opportunity-based format* of the *Additional Behaviors Data Collection Sheet*. Because Sergio occasionally engages in problematic behavior (yelling and flopping), she also decides to collect data on inappropriate behavior. After considering the different data collection formats, she selects the *frequency-based format* of the *Additional Behaviors Data Collection Sheet* because the behaviors are typically of short duration and occur infrequently enough to make it practical to collect data on each instance. She also decides to collect data on the antecedents and consequences of the behavior using the *Functional Behavior Assessment Data Sheet*.

To successfully track inappropriate behavior, Trina must establish clear definitions of the behaviors. Using the tutorial in Appendix A, Trina drafts the following definitions based on her prior observations of the behavior:

- Behavior #1: Yelling – Vocalizations above conversation level. Does not include laughing or attempts to get someone's attention from a distance.
- Behavior #2: Flopping – Falling to the floor. Does not include accidental falls or instances of sitting on the floor when appropriate for the current activity.

She plans to record a hash mark on the ***Additional Behaviors Data Collection Sheet*** each time yelling or flopping occurs during each 60-min class period. She will make a note of the date, setting (cafeteria/store), and total time of the class period (in case shorter than 60 min) where indicated on the data sheet. Figure 7.2 shows how she sets up her two data sheets.

Trina also will record antecedents and consequences for each occurrence of problem behavior on the ***Functional Behavior Assessment Data Sheet***. Because yelling and flopping tend to occur at the same time, Trina will combine them on a single data collection sheet.

Step 8: Conduct the VSSA

Trina now has everything that she needs to conduct the VSSA. Following her plan, Trina arranges the situations while working with Sergio during his regularly scheduled class periods in the cafeteria and school store. Trina completed all of the sessions in her VSSA plan in about two weeks. Although this is somewhat longer than Trina typically devotes to assessment, she felt that the VSSA provided her with valuable information to move forward with Sergio's transitional planning. Furthermore, because the VSSA was embedded within his current school activities, Sergio continued to work on his vocational goals and even learned some new tasks during those two weeks.

Step 9: Summarize and Interpret the VSSA

Once Trina completed the VSSA, she gathers all of her data sheets to summarize her observations. Starting with the ***Arranged Situations Data Sheet***, Trina summarizes the data as described in Chapter 6. An example of her calculations for one of the situations (task interrupted) is shown in Figure 7.3, and a summary of all her calculations for Sergio's responses during the VSSA is displayed in Table 7.5

Next, Trina summarizes the data on confirming statements and inappropriate behavior, collected using the ***Additional Behaviors Data Sheets***. Sergio never engaged in any confirming statements (0% of opportunities). Figure 7.4 shows the frequency data on inappropriate behavior that Trina collected during four class periods and her summary of those data.

Finally, Trina summarizes the data on the antecedents and consequences of Sergio's inappropriate behavior (yelling and/or flopping) that she collected using the ***Functional Behavior Assessment Data Sheet.*** Figure 7.5 shows the data that Trina collected and her summary of those data. Her summary, shown on the right side of the data sheet, suggests that the primary function of these behaviors is to escape tasks because the number in the box in the final row under the escape column is much higher than the numbers in the boxes under the columns for the other functions.

Trina is now ready to transfer these data summaries to Sergio's ***VSSA Results Report Form*** so that she can share the information with Sergio

Opportunity-Based Recording

Scoring: (+) correct; (-) incorrect; On-task (+) scored if no more than _____ minutes/seconds off task

Opportunities or Session #																	# correct	# of opp.	%
B1: Confirming Statements																			

Frequency Recording

Scoring: (/) for each occurrence of the behavior

Session #/Date and Time (min)						Total #	Total min	Rate (#/min)
B1: Yelling								

Session # and Time (min)						Total #	Total min	Rate (#/min)
B2: Flopping								

Figure 7.2 Trina's Additional Behaviors Data Collection Sheet for Sergio's VSSA.

Task Interrupted

Session #	2	6	8				# correct	# of opp.	%
Completes new task	+	+	+				3	3	100%
Returns to initial task	-	-	-				0	0	0%

Figure 7.3 Trina's calculations for Sergio's performance during the task-interrupted situation.

and his parents. She uses the top portion of the template report form to display the results from the Arranged Situations Data Collection Sheet and the bottom portion of the form to display the summary data from the Additional Behaviors Data Sheets. Her completed VSSA Results Report Form is displayed in Figure 7.6.

Step 10: Select the Targets for Instruction

Once Trina completes Sergio's VSSA Results Report Form, she meets with Sergio and his parents to discuss the results. In terms of his strengths, Sergio always immediately switched to a new task when Trina interrupted his current task and corrected his mistakes when Trina provided feedback. However, the form also indicated that Sergio would benefit from training on a variety of the assessed skills. Across multiple

Table 7.5 Summary of Sergio's performance during the arranged situations of the VSSA

Arranged Situations, Responses, & Percentage of Opportunities With Correct Responses

Task Interrupted
• Completes new task = 100%
• Returns to initial task = 0%

Task Completed
• Seeks supervisor 0%
• Presses finished icon = 0%

Materials Needed

• Searches for materials = 33%
• Finds materials = 0%
• Seeks assistance = 0%
• Presses help icon = 0%

Supervisor Unavailable

• N/O (no opportunities to collect data because Sergio never sought assistance)

Vague Instructions/Task Not in Repertoire

• Seeks assistance = 0%
• Presses help icon = 0%

Multiple Tasks

• Transitions = 0%

Feedback Provided

• Acknowledges feedback = 0%
• Corrects mistake = 100%

Frequency Recording

Scoring: (/) for each occurrence of the behavior

Date/Setting/Time (min)	2/16 – Store-60 min	2/20 – Café. – 60 min	2/22 – Store – 45 min	2/25 – Cafe. – 60 min	Total #	Total min	Rate (#/min)
Yelling	//	///	///	//	10	225	.04
Flopping		/	/	/	3	225	.01

Figure 7.4 Trina's data on Sergio's inappropriate behaviors during the VSSA.

Functional Behavior Assessment

Target Behavior: Yelling / Flopping	Definition: <u>Yelling</u> - Vocalizations above conversation level, not including laughing or getting someone's attention from a distance. <u>Flopping</u>: Falling to the floor, not including accidental falls or sitting on the floor when appropriate for the current activity.

Immediate Antecedent Scoring: (X) for each instance of the behavior												Total # of Instances		
												Attention	Escape	Tangible
Supervisor unavailable												0		
Ignored by others												0		
Provided feedback	X		X		X								3	
Task interrupted		X											1	
Coworker asks for assistance													0	
Given clear instruction									X				1	
Given vague instruction			X		X	X							3	
Task not in repertoire				X			X						2	
Materials needed														0
Conversing with peer												0	0	0
Denied access to items/activities														0

Immediate consequence

Given feedback/attention	X		X		X	X			X			5		
Ignored		X		X			X	X		X			5	
Task delayed or removed				X		X	X		X				4	
Provided items/activities														0
Provided break													0	0
											Totals:	5	19	0

If the highest number of instances of the target behavior were scored as **attention**, this indicates the learner most likely engages in the target behavior to access attention; this may be in the form of conversation, reprimands, or a reaction.

If the highest number of instances of the target behavior were scored as **escape**, this indicates the learner most likely engages in the target behavior to avoid work, get out of completing certain tasks, or get a break.

If the highest number of instances of the target behavior were scored as **tangible**, this indicates the learner most likely engages in the target behavior to gain access to an item or activity such as food, electronics, or personal items.

Figure 7.5 Trina's completed Functional Behavior Assessment Data Sheet for Sergio during the VSSA.

situations, Sergio did not seek assistance when needed or use his communication device to convey his needs, and he did not transition independently across tasks. As a result, he spent a considerable amount of time waiting for Trina to notice that he needed assistance and to prompt him to complete the next task. He never confirmed his understanding of instructions or acknowledged receipt of feedback.

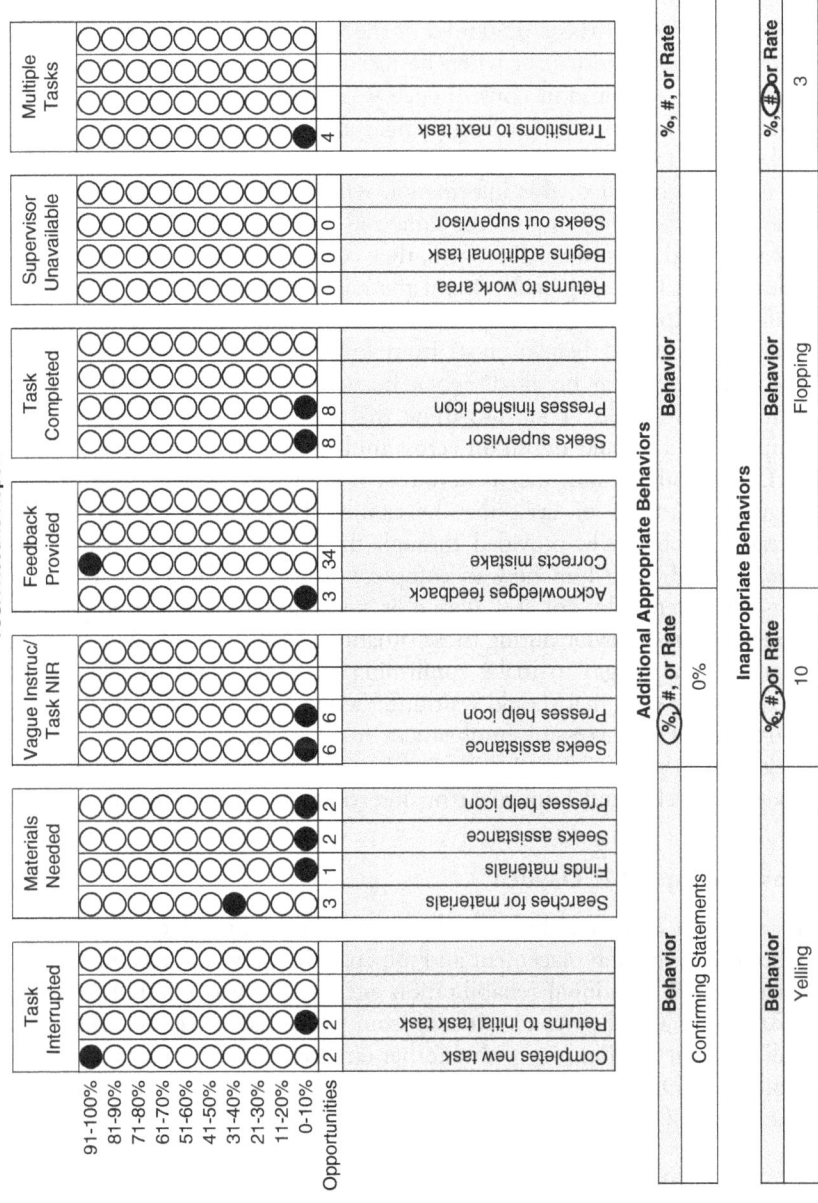

Figure 7.6 Sergio's completed VSSA Results Report Form. NIR = Not in Repertoire.

Next, Trina discusses the data collected on Sergio's yelling and flopping and also shows them the completed Functional Behavior Assessment Data Sheet. She noted that yelling occurred more often than flopping and that both typically occurred when Sergio received a task that he had never completed before (those presented in the vague-instructions and task-not-in-repertoire situations) or when he received feedback about his work on those tasks. A common consequence was a delay in having to complete those tasks, suggesting that Sergio engaged in these behaviors to escape or delay these tasks.

After sharing all of this information with Sergio and his parents, Trina then asked for their input on the skills and associated situations to prioritize for intervention. In their discussion, they considered Sergio's job preferences (cleaning and stocking shelves) and the relative importance of the different skills in helping Sergio obtain and maintain employment. They decided that Sergio would benefit most from learning to seek assistance and to communicate using his iPad® when he needs materials and when he has completed his tasks. They also think that Sergio would be a more valued employee if he could transition across multiple tasks without assistance.

On the other hand, they believe that it is unlikely Sergio will encounter vague instructions or tasks that he cannot do at his first job placement because a job coach, provided through the state's supported employment services, will teach him how to complete assigned tasks. Thus, Trina and Sergio's parents do not feel that it is necessary to target appropriate or inappropriate behavior during those situations at this time. They also decide that teaching Sergio to make confirming statements and to acknowledge feedback are skills that should wait until Sergio has acquired skills that seem most critical to successful employment (e.g., asking for help, transitioning independently across tasks). Chapter 12 will describe the steps that Trina takes to develop and implement his intervention for these skills.

Case Example #2: Dayden

Dayden is a 25-year-old man with autism and mild intellectual disabilities who is receiving job placement and job coaching services through his local, state-funded vocational rehabilitation agency. He was referred to a local ABA center after he was terminated from two consecutive jobs. Before she will consider placing him with another employer, his vocational counselor would like Dayden to receive behavior intervention services to increase the likelihood of his success on the next job placement.

Step 1: Gather Information

The ABA center's instructor, Harlow, begins the process by meeting with Dayden, his parents, and his vocational counselor to obtain information pertinent to the VSSA. Using the interview form in Appendix A, Harlow obtains the following information:

- Dayden was unable to maintain employment at a grocery store (first job placement) and a large retail store (second job placement). He was terminated from both jobs for becoming argumentative with his supervisors, particularly when he received feedback. His supervisors also reported that he would remain idle when he finished his assigned tasks or couldn't find his supervisor when he needed help. Dayden enjoys speaking with others, and people consider him to be very sociable and outgoing. However, his supervisors at the grocery store expressed concern that he would frequently engage in extended conversations with customers while he was bagging groceries, asking them inappropriate questions and sharing personal information. He did not respond appropriately to the customers' signs of disinterest in conversing with him.
- Dayden would like to work in a retail or grocery store where he can greet or assist customers, stock shelves, and bag purchases. He would prefer to work with others.
- At home, Dayden cleans his room, helps his parents prepare meals, feeds and walks the dog, and takes out the trash.
- Dayden knows how to complete basic tasks, such as folding papers, filing, alphabetizing books, folding shirts, cleaning tables, rolling silverware, bagging groceries, stocking shelves, stapling, shredding paper, and sorting objects. He knows how to search the internet, use Microsoft Word®, print documents, and count change. He does not know how to use Microsoft Excel® or Microsoft Powerpoint®. He can tell time using an analog or digital clock.
- Dayden reads and writes on an 8th-grade level.
- Dayden follows directions and is generally eager to please. However, he became argumentative with supervisors at his prior placements when he received conflicting instructions and feedback and when his supervisors told him to stop talking so much to customers.

Step 2: Select the Arranged Situations

Harlow considers the reasons that Dayden has not been successful on the job when selecting the situations to include in the VSSA. In light of potential difficulties with conflicting instructions and feedback from supervisors, remaining off-task when he needs help or doesn't know what to do, and inappropriate conversations with customers, Harlow decides to include all seven recommended situations outlined in the VSSA protocol. He also will arrange for Dayden to complete work and take breaks with other people (i.e., available peers or staff) during some of the sessions at the ABA center to assess appropriate and inappropriate conversation skills. His final list of arranged situations is displayed in Table 7.6.

Table 7.6 Dayden's arranged situations for the VSSA

Task Interrupted
Materials Needed
Vague Instructions
Task Not in Repertoire
Feedback Provided (Clear, Conflicting)
Task Completed
Supervisor Unavailable
Breaks With Others

Step 3: Select the Tasks

Because Harlow must conduct the VSSA within the context of a simulated work environment at the ABA center, he considers tasks that would be practical to arrange in this environment. He regularly includes basic tasks, such as stapling, filing, shredding, rolling silverware, cleaning rooms, folding shirts, typing, printing documents, and stuffing envelopes, in his center-based VSSAs. Harlow also decides to include stocking and bagging merchandise based on information about Dayden's preferred jobs. Next, Hayen considers tasks that would be appropriate for the vague-instructions and task-not-in-repertoire situations. Vague instructions could be delivered when assigning tasks that can be completed in multiple ways, such as alphabetizing books, folding shirts, stocking shelves, sorting objects, and filing. Harlow has learned that Dayden does not know how to use Microsoft Excel® or Microsoft Powerpoint®, and he thinks that it is unlikely Dayden knows how to laminate cards, a task that is often completed at the center. Thus, he decides to include these tasks in the VSSA for the task-not-in-repertoire situation.

Harlow's final list of tasks, along with the possible situations that he might arrange when assigning those tasks, appears in Table 7.7. Note that the VSSA protocol does not recommend interrupting any tasks that are assigned to the vague-instructions or task-not-in-repertoire situations. Harlow does not plan to have Dayden finish any tasks that are not in his repertoire due to the extensive assistance he likely would need to complete them. Harlow can arrange to provide feedback during any of the tasks and can arrange to be unavailable for any situation requiring his assistance.

Step 4: Select the Task Amounts

Harlow plans to schedule Dayden's VSSA to occur during two-hour "work shifts" across three separate days at the center (for a total of six hours), as this schedule will work best for Dayden. Harlow believes that he can complete all of the planned situations in a total of six hours as long as the tasks are not lengthy. For all tasks, he plans to assign amounts that Dayden

Table 7.7 Dayden's selected tasks for the VSSA

Tasks	Potential Arranged Situations*
Shredding	Task Interrupted, Task Completed
Stuffing envelopes	Task Interrupted, Task Completed
Stapling	Task Interrupted, Materials Needed, Task Completed
Rolling silverware	Task Interrupted, Materials Needed, Task Completed
Cleaning tables	Task Interrupted, Materials Needed, Task Completed
Put shirts on hangers	Task Interrupted, Materials Needed, Task Completed
Filing	Vague Instructions, Task Completed
Folding shirts	Vague Instructions, Task Completed
Stocking shelves	Vague Instructions, Task Completed
Alphabetizing books	Vague Instructions, Task Completed
Sorting cards	Vague Instructions, Task Completed
Creating a spreadsheet in Excel®	Task Not In Repertoire
Creating a graph in Excel	Task Not In Repertoire
Typing a document	Task Not In Repertoire
Laminating cards	Task Not In Repertoire
Creating a presentation	Task Not In Repertoire

* NOTES: Feedback can be delivered during any of Dayden's tasks; Supervisor Unavailable can be arranged for any situation requiring supervisor assistance.

likely could complete in about 15 minutes. None of Dayden's reported problems at his previous jobs seem relevant to the duration of the tasks.

Step 5: Arrange the Environment

At the ABA center, Harlow has access to several rooms that he can designate as the workroom, supervisor's office, and break room. He arranges the workroom so that it contains a work table with two chairs, a computer desk with a computer and printer, a supply cabinet, and four stackable storage shelves that he uses for stocking tasks. The work table is large enough so that Harlow can arrange for a coworker to complete tasks in the same room as Dayden during a portion of the VSSA. This will provide opportunities for Harlow to evaluate his social interactions with coworkers.

Harlow will position himself in the supervisor's office across the hall from the workroom. This will allow him to observe how Dayden performs in the absence of a supervisor's close proximity. By keeping both doors open, Harlow will be able to collect data on Dayden's performance without the assistance of another instructor, as Dayden will remain in his line of sight. When arranging the supervisor-unavailable situation, Harlow will go to another office and close the door. He will return to the workroom after a sufficient amount of time has passed for Dayden to discover that Harlow is not in his office and to respond accordingly.

Finally, Harlow arranges to use a break room down the hall, which contains several tables with chairs, a television, books, and a couch. During at least some of the breaks, Harlow will arrange for at least one person to be present in the room so that he can obtain information about his social interactions with others on the job.

Step 6: Create the Assessment Plan

Next, Harlow creates the assessment plan in Table 7.8 to help him stay organized and to ensure that he includes at least three opportunities for Dayden to experience each situation. He also is careful to document when he plans to give clear feedback versus conflicting feedback (i.e., feedback that conflicts with his initial instructions) and when a coworker will be present in the workroom or break room.

Step 7: Establish the Data Collection System

Harlow's next step is to determine how he will collect data on Dayden's performance. Harlow plans to use the ***Arranged Situations Sample Data Sheet*** discussed in Chapter 5 and provided in Appendix B because it includes all of the situations in his VSSA plan. Next, Harlow identifies other behaviors to measure by considering the behaviors discussed in Chapter 5 and the information he has obtained about Dayden's inappropriate behaviors (e.g., arguing with supervisors, engaging in inappropriate conversation with customers) and his job preferences (e.g., greeting and assisting customers). He decides to collect data on behaviors that would be incompatible with the inappropriate behaviors, as well as those that are consistent with Dayden's job preferences. This includes making confirming statements, thanking others, greeting others, and complimenting others. In addition, he will track occurrences of the reported inappropriate behavior.

Based on the recommendations in Chapter 5, Harlow will use the ***opportunity-based format*** of the ***Additional Behaviors Data Collection Sheet*** to collect data on confirming statements and thanking others, and the ***frequency-based format*** of this sheet to collect data on the remaining appropriate and inappropriate behaviors. To successfully track these behaviors, Harlow establishes the following definitions:

- Appropriate Behaviors
    - Confirming Statements. Saying "OK," "I got it," "Will do," or similar expressions to indicate understanding when given instructions.

Table 7.8 Dayden's Assessment Plan

Session	Task(s)	Arranged Situation(s)	Materials Needed

Dayden's Assessment Plan

Session	Task(s)	Arranged Situation(s)	Materials Needed
1	Roll silverware (interrupt); Shred	Task Interrupted; Task Completed	15 sets of silverware; 15 napkins; stack of paper; shredder
2	Staple	Missing Materials (staples in cabinet); Task Completed	20 sets of papers; stapler with 5 staples
3	Clean table and computer desk	Task Completed	Spray bottle; cloth
4	File	Vague Instructions; Clear Feedback	30 papers that can be filed by name or color; file box
Break (coworkers present)			
5	Create Excel spreadsheet	Task Not In Repertoire; Supervisor Unavailable	Computer; data
6	Stuff envelopes (interrupt);Shred	Task interrupted; Task Completed (coworker present)	30 letters and envelopes; Stack of paper; shredder
7	Roll silverware	Missing Materials (napkins with supervisor); Supervisor Unavailable; Task Completed	15 sets of silverware; 10 napkins
8	Laminate cards	Task Not In Repertoire	10 cards; laminating sheets; laminator
Break (coworker present)			
9	Sort cards	Vague Instructions; Clear Feedback; Task Completed	50 cards (can be sorted by animal, name, or color)
10	Clean table and computer desk	Missing Materials (cloth with supervisor) Conflicting Feedback	Spray bottle (cloth missing)
11	Fold shirts	Vague Instructions; Clear Feedback Task Completed (coworker present)	20 t-shirts
12	Create presentation	Task Not In Repertoire	Computer; print out of topic content
Break			
13	Stuff envelopes (interrupt); Put shirts on hangers	Task interrupted; Missing Materials (Hangers in cabinet); Task Completed	20 letters and envelopes; 15 shirts; 15 hangers (2 broken)
14	Staple	Task Completed Supervisor Unavailable; Conflicting Feedback	20 sets of papers
15	File	Clear Instructions Conflicting Feedback	40 letters, file box

- Greeting Others: Saying "hello," "hi," "how are you," and other similar expressions of greeting.
- Thanking Others: Saying "thanks," "thank you," "I appreciate that," and other similar expressions of gratitude.
- Complimenting Others: Saying 'I like _____, "It's great how you _____," or a similar expression of admiration in reference to the person's behavior (e.g., completing high-quality work) or an item in the person's possession (e.g., article of clothing, accessory).

- Inappropriate Behaviors

  - Arguing: Expressing disagreement or contradicting someone in a negative tone of voice.
  - Inappropriate Conversation: Asking personal questions or conveying information of a personal nature; initiating a conversation about non-work related topics, unless he and the conversation partner are on a scheduled break.

He plans to record whether Dayden makes a confirming statement whenever he is given a task instruction and whether he thanks others whenever someone assists him or honors a request (opportunity-based recording). Harlow will record a hash mark when Dayden engages in each of the remaining behaviors during each two-hour appointment (frequency-based recording). Finally, Harlow also will collect data on the antecedents and consequences of Dayden's argumentative statements using the **Functional Behavior Assessment Data Sheet**. Figure 7.7 shows how he sets up the **Additional Behaviors Data Collection Sheet**.

Step 8: Conduct the VSSA

Harlow now has everything that he needs to conduct the VSSA. However, as recommended in Chapter 4, Harlow still needs to consider how he will respond to Dayden's inappropriate behaviors if they occur during the VSSA. Although Harlow has learned from Chapter 4 that he should react to Dayden's arguing and inappropriate conversation in the same way that supervisors, coworkers, and customers did on his prior jobs, Harlow was not able to obtain this information prior to the assessment. Thus, Harlow decides to follow the guidance provided in Chapter 4 for this situation. He will provide as little visible reaction as possible while continuing with the assessment. For example, if Dayden argues when told to correct his mistakes, Harlow will not engage in the argument and will simply tell him again to correct his work before returning to his office across the hall from Dayden's workroom. In the case of inappropriate conversation with peers during breaks or work sessions, Harlow will collect data on the behavior without interfering or prompting the peers to respond in any particular manner.

Opportunity-Based Recording

Scoring: (+) correct; (−) incorrect:

Date														# correct	# of opp.	%
Opportunities or Session #																
Confirming Statements																

Scoring: (+) correct; (−) incorrect

Date														# correct	# of opp.	%
Opportunities or Session #																
Thanking Others																

Frequency Recording

Scoring: (/) for each occurrence of the behavior

Date/Session #/Time (min)		Total #	Total min	Rate (#/min)
Greeting				
Rate (#/min):				
Complimenting				
Rate (#/min):				
Arguing				
Rate (#/min):				
Inappropriate Conversation				
Rate (#/min):				

Figure 7.7 Harlow's Additional Behaviors Data Collection Sheet for Dayden's VSSA.

At the start of each two-hour appointment, Harlow shows Dayden the location of the workroom, supply cabinet, supervisor's office, and break room. He then follows his VSSA plan and completes it in three appointments.

Step 9: Summarize and Interpret the VSSA

Once Hayden completes the VSSA, he gathers all of the data sheets to summarize the observations. He starts with the *Arranged Situations Data Sheet*. A summary of those data, conducted as described in Chapter 6, produced the results in Table 7.9.

Next, Harlow summarizes the data on Dayden's appropriate behaviors, collected using the opportunity- and frequency-based formats of the *Additional Behaviors Data Collection Sheet.* When summarizing data on the opportunity-based sheet, Harlow found that Dayden never confirmed his understanding of instructions (0% of opportunities) and rarely thanked others (12% of opportunities). From the frequency-based sheet, Harlow determined that Dayden frequently greeted others (11 times) but never delivered any compliments, and he often engaged in argumentative and inappropriate conversational statements (25 and 13 times, respectively) across the VSSA.

Harlow then summarizes the data on the antecedents and consequences of Dayden's argumentative statements that he collected using the *Functional Behavior Assessment Data Sheet.* His summary on the final

Table 7.9 Summary of Dayden's performance during the arranged situations of the VSSA

Arranged Situations, Responses, & Percentage of Opportunities With Correct Responses

Task Interrupted
• Completes new task = 33%
• Returns to initial task = 0%

Materials Needed
• Searches for materials = 25%
• Finds materials = 100%
• Seeks assistance = 100%
• Requests help = 100%

Vague Instructions/Task Not in Repertoire
• Seeks assistance = 100%
• Requests help = 100%

Feedback Provided
• Acknowledges feedback = 0%
• Asks for clear feedback = 0%
• Confirms understanding = 0%
• Corrects mistake = 16%

Task Completed
• Seeks supervisor = 100%
• Requests help = 100%

Supervisor Unavailable
• Returns to room = 100%
• Seeks other work = 0%
• Seeks out supervisor again = 0%

Breaks
• Returns on time = 0%

page of the data sheet, as shown in Figure 7.8, confirmed that Dayden primarily argued when given feedback. Because Harlow purposefully ignored all instances of argumentative statements and returned to his office after repeating the instructions once, the most commonly occurring consequence was delay or removal of a task. Hayden's summary shows strong support for an escape function. Note that the numbers shown in the summary (right column) section of the sheet include instances of behavior and events that occurred on prior, filled pages of the data sheet.

Functional Behavior Assessment

Target Behavior: Arguing	Definition: Expressing disagreement or contradicting someone in a negative tone of voice

Immediate Antecedent	Scoring: (X) for each instance of the behavior										Attention	Escape	Tangible
											Total # of Instances		
Supervisor unavailable											0		
Ignored by others											0		
Provided feedback	X	X		X		X	X	X				14	
Task interrupted			X						X			3	
Coworker asks for assistance												0	
Given clear instruction												0	
Vague instruction												0	
Task not in repertoire					X			X				2	
Materials needed													0
Conversing with peer					X						1	1	1
Denied access to items/activities													0

Immediate consequence

											Attention	Escape	Tangible
Given feedback/attention											1		
Ignored	X	X	X	X	X	X	X	X	X	X		25	
Task delayed or removed	X	X	X	X	X	X	X	X	X	X		25	
Provided items/activities													0
Provided break												0	0
Totals:											2	70	1

If the highest number of instances of the target behavior were scored as **attention**, this indicates the learner most likely engages in the target behavior to access attention; this may be in the form of conversation, reprimands, or a reaction.

If the highest number of instances of the target behavior were scored as **escape**, this indicates the learner most likely engages in the target behavior to avoid work, get out of completing certain tasks, or get a break.

If the highest number of instances of the target behavior were scored as **tangible**, this indicates the learner most likely engages in the target behavior to gain access to an item or activity such as food, electronics, or personal items.

Figure 7.8 Harlow's completed Functional Behavior Assessment Data Sheet for Dayden during the VSSA.

Step 10: Select the Targets for Instruction

Harlow meets with Dayden, his parents, and his vocational counselor to review Dayden's completed **VSSA Results Report Form**. As shown in Figure 7.9, Harlow uses the top portion of the template report form to display the results from the Arranged Situations Data Collection Sheet and the bottom portion of the form to display the summary data from the Additional Behaviors Data Sheets.

Harlow begins by summarizing Dayden's strengths. Harlow notes that Dayden worked hard and seemed motivated to perform well at the Center. He was friendly and greeted people frequently when the opportunity arose. Dayden always immediately switched to a new task when Harlow interrupted his current task, and he requested help from his supervisor when needed.

In terms of skills that needed improvement, Dayden remained off-task for long periods of time when Harlow was not available to help him. Dayden would simply wait in the work or break room rather than switching to other available tasks, and he never checked back to see if Harlow had returned to his office. Dayden also did not respond appropriately when he received feedback, regardless of whether it was consistent or inconsistent (i.e., conflicted) with Harlow's initial instructions. He would typically argue with Harlow about the best way to do the task and refuse to re-do the work as instructed. Harlow rarely observed Dayden thanking or complimenting others. Finally, while on break, Dayden always initiated and maintained conversations with peers, but he sometimes asked questions of a personal nature that would be inappropriate to ask coworkers (e.g., "Are your parents divorced?" "Do you have a boyfriend?"). He also never returned from his breaks at the designated ending time.

Next, Harlow asked Dayden, his parents, and the vocational counselor for their input on the skills and associated situations to prioritize for intervention. In their discussion, they considered Dayden's job preferences (greeting or assisting customers, stocking shelves, and bagging purchases in a retail store) and the reasons that he was not successful at his prior job placements (arguing with supervisors, remaining off-task when he couldn't get help, engaging in inappropriate conversation with customers). Harlow discussed the importance of targeting appropriate responses that would replace inappropriate behavior. By the end of the meeting, they decided that Dayden should begin by learning how to (1) respond appropriately to feedback, (2) complete other work when his supervisor was not available to assist, and (3) engage in appropriate conversation with customers and coworkers. Chapter 12 provides a detailed description of the steps that Harlow takes to develop and implement the VSSI for these skills.

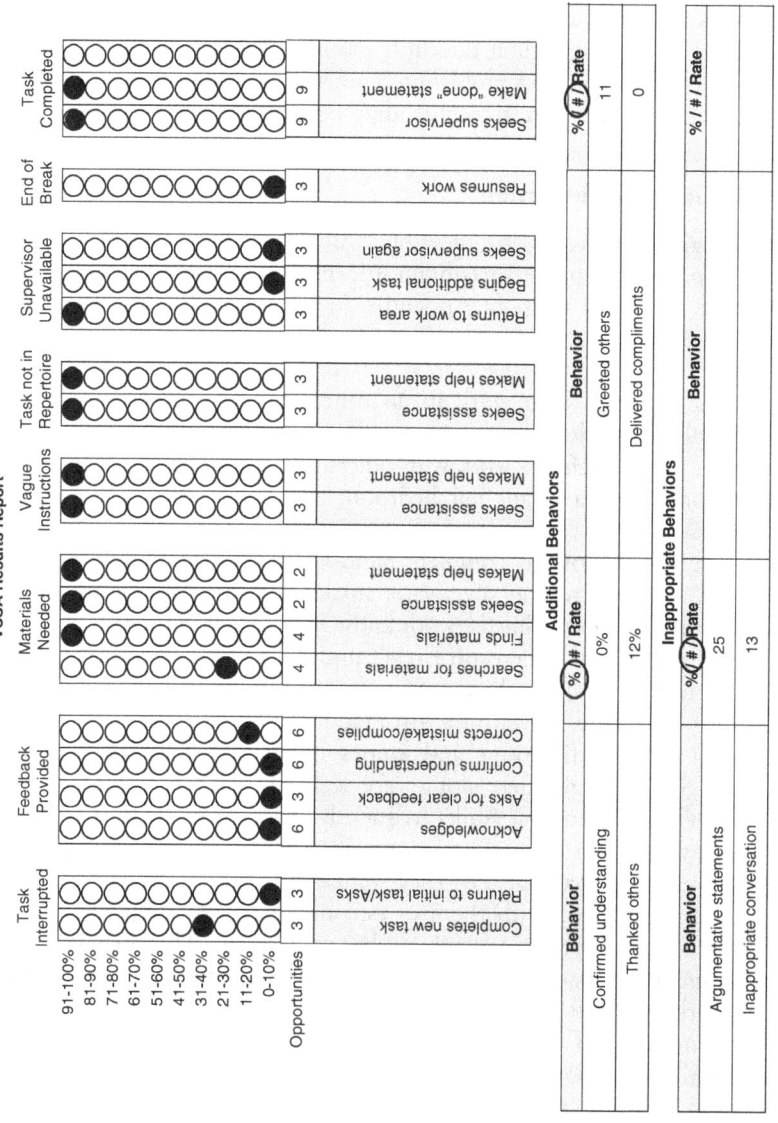

Figure 7.9 Dayden's completed VSSA Results Report Form.

Case Example #3 – Anika

Anika is a 28-year-old woman with autism and moderate intellectual abilities who is receiving job training services through her local VR office. She has volunteered at her church and a local animal shelter but has never been employed. She is currently receiving job training at a thrift shop for 4 hours each week with the assistance of a job coach provided by the VR office. Although she is doing well at the thrift shop, her job coach, Jaycee, would like to assess her social and problem-solving skills to determine if she needs any further training before recommending her for job placement services.

Step 1: Gather Information

Jaycee begins the process by meeting with Anika, her supervisor at the thrift shop, and her parents to obtain information pertinent to the VSSA. Using the interview form in Appendix A, Jaycee obtains the following information:

- Anika would like to work in an office, a movie theatre, or at an animal shelter doing a variety of different tasks.
- Anika would prefer to work with others, but she is fine working alone.
- At home, Anika cleans her bedroom and helps her family prepare meals.
- Anika knows how to complete basic tasks, such as folding clothes, filing, stapling, rolling silverware, stocking shelves, shredding paper, and sorting objects. She does not know how to search the Internet, use Microsoft Word®, Microsoft Excel®, and Microsoft Powerpoint®, print documents, or count change. She can tell time using a digital clock.
- Anika reads and writes on a 4th-grade level.
- Anika follows directions and enjoys being told that she is doing well. She generally gets along very well with others. However, her supervisor reports that Anika frequently asks coworkers to share their food with her or to lend her money so that she can get a snack from the vending machine. If they refuse Anika's requests, she will continue to plead with them or become angry. As such, they often give her food or money when she requests it. This behavior has prevented Anika from developing good relationships with her coworkers, who often avoid her due to these requests. Anika continues to do this even though her supervisor has spoken to her several times about it.
- Jaycee has noticed that Anika rarely orients toward others during conversation, regardless of whether she is speaking or listening to someone else. She generally will look away, with her body turned at least 180 degrees away from the person. However, she typically smiles while engaging in conversation and uses a friendly tone.

Step 2: Select the Arranged Situations

Jaycee decides to include all seven recommended situations outlined in the VSSA protocol, as she would like to identify a variety of social and problem-solving skills that Anika may need to target prior to job placement. In consideration of her job preferences, Jaycee decides to include supervisor-needs-assistance, multiple-task, and instructed-to-relay-information situations because they seem relevant to Anika's desired job placements and Jaycee has not had opportunities to observe Anika in those situations at the thrift shop. Jaycee consults the quick reference tables for these situations provided in Appendix A of this book when deciding how to set up these situations and selecting the responses to target in these situations. For the supervisor-needs-assistance situation, Jaycee or the thrift supervisor will spill items or attempt to lift/move heavy boxes near Anika while she is working to determine if she will offer unsolicited help to others. For the multiple-task situation, the supervisor will instruct Anika to complete three tasks in a particular sequence. For the relay-information situation, Jaycee or the supervisor will ask Anika to convey spoken or written information to another person at the thrift shop. Jaycee will have opportunities throughout the assessment to observe Anika's inappropriate requests for food or money from her coworkers. Her final list of arranged situations is displayed in Table 7.10.

Step 3: Select the Tasks

With the assistance of the thrift shop supervisor, Jaycee plans to conduct the VSSA while Anika is working at the shop. Her regular responsibilities include sorting the donations, hanging and folding clothes, and organizing the merchandise on the shelves. Jaycee also considered tasks that Anika might complete at her desired future job placements (office, movie theatre, animal shelter) and that Anika could also complete at the thrift shop. After speaking with the shop supervisor, Jaycee selected some

Table 7.10 Jaycee's arranged situations for Anika's VSSA

Task Interrupted
Materials Needed
Vague Instructions
Task Not in Repertoire
Feedback Provided (Clear, Vague, Conflicting)
Task Completed
Supervisor Unavailable
Supervisor Needs Assistance
Multiple Tasks
Instructed to Relay Information

tasks that Anika might complete at an office, movie theatre, or animal shelter (e.g., filing, stapling, shredding, sweeping, cleaning).

Jaycee necessarily needs to consider new and difficult tasks to include in the vague-instructions and task-not-in-repertoire situations. Vague instructions could be delivered when assigning new tasks that could be completed in multiple ways, such as stocking new shelving areas at the thrift shop, alphabetizing books, sorting objects, and filing. She learned that Anika does not know how to complete computer-related tasks or count change, both of which she could arrange at the thrift shop.

Jaycee's final list of tasks and potential arranged situations appear in Table 7.11. Jaycee does not plan to have Anika finish any tasks that are not in her repertoire due to the extensive assistance she likely would need to complete them. If Anika correctly asks for help with these difficult tasks, Jaycee will say, "Thanks for asking but I'd like you to do something else now." Jaycee or the supervisor can arrange to provide feedback during any of the tasks and can arrange to be unavailable for any situation requiring their assistance.

Table 7.11 Anika's selected tasks for the VSSA

Tasks	Potential Arranged Situations[*]
Shredding	Task Interrupted, Task Completed
Folding shirts	Task Interrupted, Task Completed
Hanging shirts	Task Interrupted, Materials Needed, Task Completed
Stapling	Task Interrupted, Materials Needed, Task Completed
Sweeping floor	Task Interrupted, Materials Needed, Task Completed
Cleaning chairs	Task Interrupted, Materials Needed, Task Completed
Mopping floor	Task Interrupted, Materials Needed, Task Completed
Filing	Vague Instructions, Task Completed
Sorting new items	Vague Instructions, Task Completed
Stocking new shelves	Vague Instructions, Task Completed
Alphabetizing books	Vague Instructions, Task Completed
Creating a spreadsheet	Task Not In Repertoire
Searching Internet for information	Task Not In Repertoire
Typing a document	Task Not In Repertoire
Counting money in cash register	Task Not In Repertoire
Creating a presentation	Task Not In Repertoire

[*] NOTES: Feedback can be delivered during any of Anika's tasks; Supervisor Unavailable can be arranged for any situation requiring supervisor assistance. Multiple-task situation will be arranged by assigning three tasks from the list at one time.

Step 4: Select the Task Amounts

Jaycee plans to conduct Anika's VSSA during her shifts at the thrift shop. Anika typically works two-hour shifts, two days per week. The shop supervisor is available to assist during the first hour of each shift, so Jaycee will serve as the supervisor during the second hour. Jaycee believes that she can complete all of the planned situations in about two weeks. For all but Anika's regular tasks at the shop, Jaycee will assign amounts that Anika likely could complete in about 10 minutes.

Step 5: Arrange the Environment

Next, Jaycee considers the thrift shop environment and whether it may be beneficial to alter aspects of it during the VSSA. In terms of the work locations, Anika typically sorts donations in the back room, folds and hangs shirts at the front of the shop, and organizes shelves in the household goods section. Anika is not familiar with the supply closet, as Jaycee and the shop supervisor typically provide what she needs on her shift. Thus, Jaycee will ensure that some of the items for the materials-needed situation are available in the supply cabinet, and she plans to show Anika the supply cabinet before she begins the VSSA.

Jaycee next considers the supervisor's location. The shop supervisor typically works alongside Anika when Jaycee is not present unless the supervisor has to wait on customers. When Jaycee is present, the supervisor typically remains in her office, supervises other staff, or assists customers. Jaycee would like to observe Anika's performance when she isn't given so much assistance. Thus, she identifies a location in the back room and in the shop where either she or the supervisor can remain distanced from Anika but still observe her. She plans to sit at a table or desk and pretend to be busy with something else. Before giving Anika her assigned task(s), Jaycee and the supervisor will point out their planned location and remind Anika to let them know if she needs anything. During the supervisor-unavailable situation, Jaycee will pretend to have a conversation on her cell phone and ignore any of Anika's attempts to gain her attention at that time. The shop supervisor will close her office door and pretend to have a meeting.

Step 6: Create the Assessment Plan

Next, Jaycee creates the assessment plan in Table 7.12 to stay organized and ensure that she includes at least three opportunities for Anika to experience each situation. She is also careful to document when she plans to arrange for a supervisor to need assistance and when she plans to ask Anika to relay information to another staff person or coworker. Anika typically does not take any breaks during her short shifts at the thrift store, so Jaycee does not include them in the plan.

Table 7.12 Anika's Assessment Plan

Anika's Assessment Plan			
Session	Task(s)	Arranged Situation(s)	Materials Needed
1	Fold shirts (interrupt); Shred	Task Interrupted; Task Completed	30 shirts; stack of paper; shredder
2	Sweep floor; Clean tables; Mop floor	Multiple Tasks; Materials Needed (broom in cabinet); Task Completed	Broom (missing); mop; bucket; spray bottle; ceaner; sponge
3	Relay info	Relay Information (to supervisor's assistant)	Written info (Inventory List)
4	File	Vague Instructions Clear Feedback	30 papers that can be filed by name or donation date; file box
5	Create Excel spreadsheet	Task Not In Repertoire Supervisor Unavailable	Computer; data
6	Hang shirts (interrupt); Staple	Task Interrupted; Materials Needed (staples with supervisor); Task Completed	40 shirts; 30 packets; stapler with 10 staples
7	Count money in register	Task Not in Repertoire; Supervisor Unavailable;	Cash register with paper money and coins
8	Sort donations	Supervisor in Need of Assistance (moving boxes from unloading area)	5 boxes
9	Stock new area	Vague Instructions; Vague Feedback; Task Completed	2 boxes of donated items
10	Clean chairs; Shred; Hang shirts	Multiple Tasks Materials Needed (hangers in cabinet) Conflicting Feedback (cleaning task)	Cloth (spray bottle missing); a stack of paper; 25 shirts and 20 hangers
11	Fold shirts (interrupt); Sort donations	Task Interrupted; Task Completed	20 t-shirts; 3 boxes of donations
12	Create presentation	Task Not In Repertoire; Supervisor in Need of Assistance (drops stack of folded shirts nearby)	Computer; print out of topic content; a stack of folded shirts
13	Alphabetize books	Vague Instructions; Supervisor Unavailable; Vague Feedback; Task Completed	30 books
14	Relay info	Relay Information (to Anika)	Written Info (holiday schedule)
15	Staple; Shred; Sweep Floor	Multiple Tasks Task Completed	20 sets of papers; stapler; broom, dustpan
16	Type document	Task Not in Repertoire Clear Feedback; Supervisor in Need of Assistance (spills box of donations nearby)	Document; Box of donations
17	Relay info	Relay info to thrift shop supervisor	Vocal Info (schedule for next week)

Step 7: Establish the Data Collection System

Jaycee next determines how she will collect data on Anika's performance. She will use the *Arranged Situations Template Data Sheet* as she plans to include situations that do not appear on the sample version. Jaycee also identifies two other behaviors that she believes would be important to track for Anika. As noted under Step 1, Anika often asks her coworkers for food or money, and she may persist in asking or become argumentative if they do not honor her requests. She also generally does not orient towards others when conversing.

Jaycee will use the *opportunity-based format* of the *Additional Behaviors Data Collection Sheet* to establish her data collection system for orienting because this behavior can only occur when Anika is engaged with someone else. She defines orienting as "face positioned toward conversation partner during verbal exchanges, except when visually attending to relevant task materials." Thus, each time Anika is engaged in a conversational exchange with someone else, Jaycee will score whether or not Anika is oriented towards the person.

Jaycee will use the *frequency-based format* of the *Additional Behaviors Data Collection Sheet* to collect data on requests for food or money from others. Each time that Anika either asks someone to share their food or to loan her change, she will place a hash mark on the data sheet. This will include any repeated requests following a coworker's refusal to honor the request. Figure 7.10 shows her Additional Behaviors Data Collection Sheet.

Step 8: Conduct the VSSA

Jaycee now has everything that she needs to conduct the VSSA. Before she begins, Jaycee informs Anika that she may be getting different tasks at the thrift shop in addition to her normal responsibilities. She also shows Anika the supply cabinet and informs her that she should obtain the materials that she needs to complete her work. As noted previously, the thrift shop supervisor is only available to assist during the first hour of each shift. Thus, during the first hour of each shift, Jaycee instructs the shop supervisor on how to present each of the planned work sessions while Jaycee collects data on Anika's performance. During the second hour, Jaycee serves as the supervisor and data collector. Jaycee requires about three weeks (six work shifts) to complete all of the sessions in her relatively lengthy VSSA plan. Although this may seem lengthy for an assessment, Jaycee felt that the VSSA provided her with valuable information to help prepare Anika for job placement services. Moreover, Jaycee conducted the VSSA within the context of Anika's current job-training activities, so Anika continued to work on her vocational goals and even experienced some new job responsibilities during this time.

Opportunity-Based Recording

Scoring: (+) correct; (-) incorrect

Date																# correct	# of opp.	%
Opportunities or Session #																		
Orienting																		

Frequency Recording

Scoring: (/) for each occurrence of the behavior

Date/Session #/Time (min)						Total #	Total min	Rate (#/min)
Requesting food or money								
Rate (#/min):								

Figure 7.10 Jaycee's Additional Behaviors Data Collection Sheet for Anika's VSSA.

Step 9: Summarize and Interpret the VSSA

Once Jaycee completes the VSSA, she gathers all of the data sheets to summarize the observations. She starts with the *Arranged Situations Data Sheet.* A summary of those data, conducted as described in Chapter 6, produced the results in Table 7.13.

Next, Jaycee summarizes the data on orienting and inappropriate requests from the *Additional Behaviors Data Collection Sheets.* Her calculations indicate that Anika oriented towards her conversation partner during just 10% of her interactions with others and that she requested either food or money from her coworkers a total of 8 times during the assessment period, which was conducted across 6 work shifts at the shop.

Step 10: Select the Targets for Instruction

Jaycee transfers the results to the *VSSA Results Report Form*, a portion of which is shown in Figure 7.11, and then meets with Anika, her supervisor at the thrift shop, and her parents to review the outcomes of the assessment. As she reviews the form with the group, Jaycee notes that Anika always asked for help when she needed materials and had

Table 7.13 Summary of Anika's performance during the arranged situations of the VSSA; N/O = no opportunity for Anika to engage in the response

---

Arranged Situations, Responses, & Percentage of Opportunities With Correct Responses

---

Task Interrupted
• Completes new task = 100%
• Returns to initial task = 100%

Materials Needed
• Searches for materials = 0%
• Finds materials = N/A
• Seeks assistance = 100%
• Requests help = 100%

Vague Instructions/Task Not in Repertoire
• Seeks assistance = 0%
• Requests help = 0%

Supervisor Unavailable
• Returns to room = 100%
• Seeks other work = 67%
• Seeks supervisor again = 0%

Task Completed
• Seeks supervisor = 100%
• Requests help = 100%

Feedback Provided
• Acknowledges feedback = 0%
• Asks for clear feedback = 0%
• Confirms understanding = 0%
• Corrects mistake = 100%

Multiple Tasks
• Correct transitions = 83%

Relay Information
• Seeks Person = 100%
• Relays Information Correctly = 100%
• Returns to Work = 66%

Supervisor Needs Assistance
• Offers assistance = 0%
• Provides assistance = 0%
• Responds to gratitude – N/O
• Returns to work – N/O

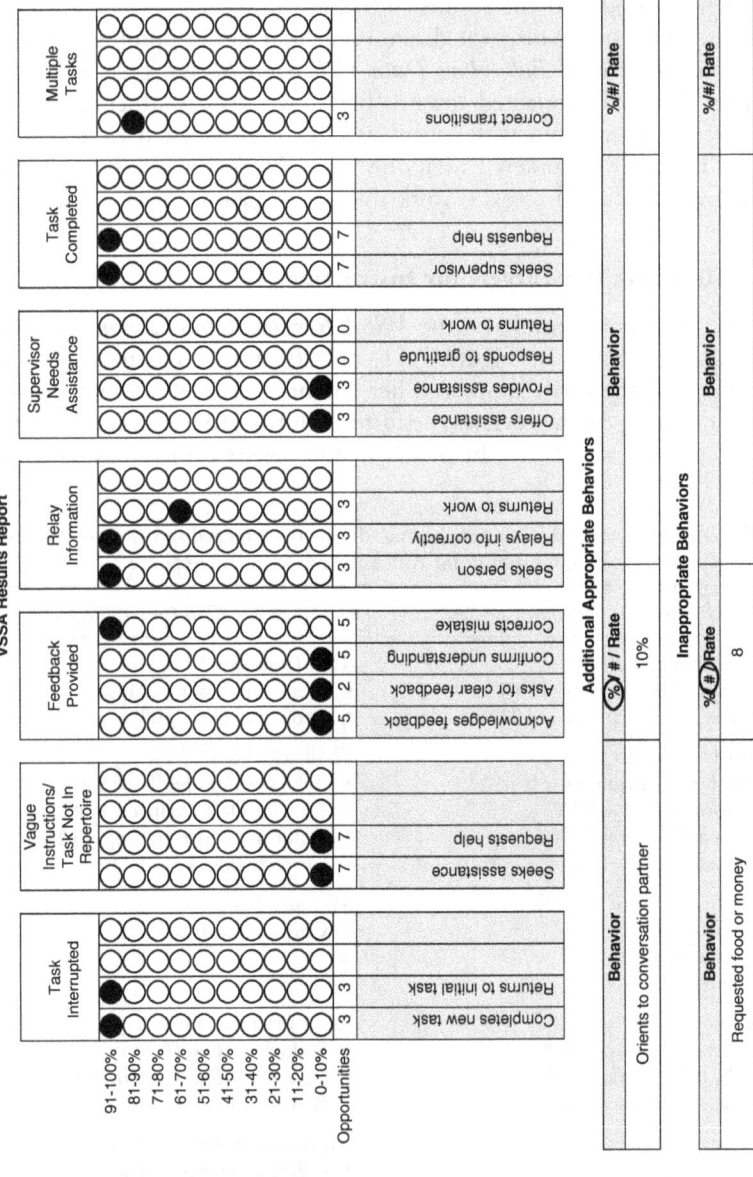

Figure 7.11 A portion of Anika's completed VSSA Results Report Form.

completed her work, and she almost always transitioned independently across multiple tasks. She also always corrected her work when given feedback. Anika's additional strengths included responding appropriately when a task was interrupted and staying on task even when her supervisor was unavailable to assist her. Finally, she accurately relayed information to other people at the thrift shop when asked.

Jaycee then described potential areas for improvement. She noted that Anika never asked for help when given vague instructions or a task that was not in her repertoire. Although she always corrected her mistakes in response to feedback, she never acknowledged the feedback, requested clearer feedback when needed, or confirmed her understanding of the feedback. Anika also requested food or money from her coworkers at least once during each shift at the shop. On two occasions, she repeated her request in an angry tone of voice when the coworker stated that they did not want to share their food. Finally, she rarely oriented towards others during interactions and never offered or provided unsolicited assistance to the supervisor when the supervisor clearly needed help.

Jaycee, Anika, her parents, and the shop supervisor then discussed which skills and behaviors to prioritize for intervention in light of the wide variety of Anika's preferred job placements (office, movie theatre, animal shelter) and the problematic behavior identified during the assessment (e.g., inappropriate requests). They decided that Anika would benefit by learning how to ask for help with tasks that she did not know how to complete so that she could excel when first starting a new job. They also felt that Anika would benefit from instruction on skills that would improve her relationships with coworkers and customers. This included how to recognize when a supervisor needed help, how to ensure that she brought everything that she would need during her work shifts (particularly, snacks and money), and how to respond appropriately when someone refuses a request. Finally, when Jaycee discussed the benefits of orienting towards others, Anika stated that she had always wanted to learn this skill.

Chapter 12 provides a detailed description of the steps that Jaycee takes to develop and implement the VSSI for these skills.

Case Example #4: Michelle

Michelle is a 19-year-old woman with autism, ADHD, and mild cognitive impairment who has never been employed. She received special education services while in school but no vocational training. She has no work or volunteer experience. Michelle lives with her parents in a very rural area of their state where there are no providers who work with the vocational rehabilitation agency. Michelle and her family would like assistance in determining if she is ready to seek competitive employment. However, they have requested telehealth services via a videoconferencing platform like Zoom™ because of the parents' current work schedule and their distance from qualified providers. Bella, a job coach who works with an organization in their state, has agreed to provide remote services.

Step 1: Gather Information

Bella begins the process by meeting remotely with Michelle, her mother, and Michelle's vocational counselor to obtain information pertinent to the VSSA and remote services. Bella obtains the following information:

- Michelle's mother has a laptop with a webcam and high-speed Internet access. The family's kitchen has good lighting and adequate space for a large table to serve as a work area for Michelle.
- Michelle is willing to work with Bella through the laptop and has experience receiving and following instructions delivered by others in a remote format.
- Michelle would like to work in a small retail or department store where she can assist customers, organize products, and work the cash register.
- At home, Michelle cleans her bedroom and bathroom, washes the dishes, and makes her own meals.
- Michelle knows how to complete basic tasks, such as folding papers, filing, alphabetizing books, stapling, shredding paper, and sorting objects. She also knows how to count change and use Microsoft Word®. She has never rolled silverware, stocked shelves, or used Microsoft Excel® or Microsoft Powerpoint®. She can tell time using a digital clock.
- Michelle reads and writes on a 6th-grade level.
- Michelle follows directions and is generally eager to please. However, she sometimes complains and protests when asked to complete tasks even though she will eventually complete them, particularly if her mother ignores the behavior. She also sometimes asks strangers or brief acquaintances inappropriately personal questions.

Step 2: Select the Arranged Situations

Bella considers the information obtained in Step 1 and the potential constraints of remote services. Bella would like to include all seven recommended situations outlined in the VSSA protocol to obtain data on a variety of social and problem-solving skills that Michelle may need to improve prior to job placement. Bella has successfully arranged these situations via telehealth with prior clients. In consideration of Michelle's preference for a retail job, Bella also decides to include the multiple-task situation. Her final list of arranged situations is displayed in Table 7.14.

Table 7.14 Michelle's arranged situations for the VSSA

Task Interrupted
Materials Needed
Vague Instructions
Task Not in Repertoire
Feedback Provided (Vague)
Task Completed
Supervisor Unavailable
Multiple Tasks

Step 3: Select the Tasks

Bella considers tasks that would be practical for Michelle's mother to arrange in the home and that would be appropriate for all of the planned situations. In a follow-up phone call, Michelle's mother confirms that she has paper, envelopes, a stapler, a shredder, silverware, napkins, cleaner, a broom, shirts, books, and currency (coins and dollar bills) that Bella can use to complete the assessment. Michelle'sfinal list of tasks, along with the possible situations that Bella might arrange when assigning those tasks, appears in Table 7.15.

Step 4: Select the Task Amounts

Bella plans to conduct Michelle's VSSA during one-hour telehealth appointments with the assistance of Michelle's mother. In consideration of

Table 7.15 Michelle's selected tasks for the VSSA

Tasks	Potential Arranged Situations*
Shredding	Task Interrupted, Task Completed
Stuffing envelopes	Task Interrupted, Materials Needed, Task Completed
Stapling	Task Interrupted, Materials Needed, Task Completed
Sweeping floor	Task Interrupted, Materials Needed, Task Completed
Rolling silverware	Vague Instructions, Materials Needed, Task Completed
Folding shirts	Vague Instructions, Task Completed
Alphabetizing books	Vague Instructions, Task Completed
Creating a spreadsheet in Excel®	Task Not In Repertoire
Creating a graph in Excel	Task Not In Repertoire
Creating a presentation	Task Not In Repertoire

* NOTES: Feedback can be delivered during any of the tasks; Supervisor Unavailable can be arranged for any situation requiring supervisor assistance. Up to three tasks may be assigned for the Multiple-Task situation.

the family's time, Bella has agreed to complete the assessment in just three appointments. She believes that she can complete all of the planned situations in a total of three hours as long as the tasks are not lengthy. For all tasks, she plans to assign amounts that Bella likely could complete in no more than 10 minutes

Step 5: Arrange the Environment

Bella's goal is to arrange a simulated work situation in Michelle's home, during which Michelle will receive instructions and feedback from Bella (her supervisor) via Zoom™. During the initial appointment with Michelle and her mother, Bella identifies the family's kitchen as the most viable location for the assessment due to the size of the room, its lighting, and the availability of a large table. During a separate telehealth appointment with Michelle's mother prior to the assessment, Bella determines the best placement of the laptop that will enable her to view Michelle throughout the assessment. Michelle's mother will place the necessary task materials on a nearby counter, so that Michelle can easily access them when Bella instructs her to complete tasks. For computer-related tasks, Bella will send links to any needed materials via the chat feature of Zoom™ and will instruct Michelle to share her screen so that Bella can view her work.

Bella wants to observe how Michelle will perform without the continuous monitoring of a supervisor. To that end, Bella will mute her audio and video feed after giving the instructions for each task. She will tell Michelle that she has other work to do but that Bella can call out if she needs anything. For the supervisor unavailable situation, Bella will not immediately respond when Michelle calls out for assistance.

For each appointment, Michelle's mother will help Michelle set up the equipment and connect to Zoom™ and assist with troubleshooting if Michelle encounters any technical problems. Otherwise, Michelle's mother will remain in her bedroom during the assessment.

Step 6: Create the Assessment Plan

Next, Bella creates the assessment plan in Table 7.16. Due to the abbreviated time for the VSSA, Bella plans to arrange the task-interrupted and multiple-task situations just two times during the assessment. In addition, Bella must consider how best to arrange the materials-needed situation in light of the remote modality and location of the assessment (home). She will ensure that Michelle either runs out of materials or is missing materials needed to complete certain tasks by telling Michelle's mother what to place on the kitchen counter at the start of each appointment. If Michelle lets Bella know that she needs more materials to complete an assigned task, Bella will just tell her to move on to the next task. However, Bella considers the possibility that Michelle may search

Table 7.16 Michelle's VSSA Plan

Michelle's Assessment Plan

Session	Task(s)	Arranged Situation(s)	Materials Needed
1	Stuff envelopes (interrupt); Shred	Task Interrupted; Task Completed	10 sets of paper and envelopes; a stack of paper; shredder
2	Staple	Materials Needed; Task Completed	10 sets of papers; stapler with 5 staples
3	Clean table	Vague Feedback; Task Completed	cleaner, cloth
4	Roll silverware	Vague Instructions; Vague Feedback	10 sets of silverware and napkins
5	Create Excel spreadsheet	Task Not In Repertoire; Supervisor Unavailable	Computer; data
6	Sweep floor; Shred; Staple	Multiple Tasks; Task Completed	Broom; dustpan; Stack of paper; shredder; 10 sets of papers; stapler
7	Roll silverware	Materials Needed; Supervisor Unavailable;	10 sets of silverware; 5 napkins
8	Create Excel graph	Task Not In Repertoire	Data
9	Fold shirts	Vague Instructions; Vague Feedback; Task Completed	10 shirts
10	Clean table	Materials Needed; Vague Feedback	Spray bottle; cloth (missing)
12	Create presentation	Task Not In Repertoire	Computer; print out of topic content
13	Alphabetize books	Vague Instructions; Vague Feedback	15 books
14	Shred (interrupt); Sweep floor	Task Interrupted; Task Completed	Stack of paper, shredder Broom, dustpan
15	Staple	Task Completed; Supervisor Unavailable; Vague Feedback	20 sets of papers
16	Stuff envelopes; Fold shirts; Alphabetize books	Multiple Task	10 letters and envelopes; 10 shirts; 10 books

for the needed materials elsewhere in the home before letting Bella know about the problem. She is prepared to document if this occurs (with the mother's assistance); however, Bella will not consider Michelle's failure to do so as an incorrect response to the situation. Finally, Bella will ensure that Michelle always has access to extra task materials for certain tasks (none assigned to the materials-needed situation) so that she has an opportunity to work on another task when the supervisor is unavailable.

Step 7: Establish the Data Collection System

Bella will create her own data sheet using the ***Arranged Situations Template Data Sheet*** because, as noted previously, she plans to include a multiple-task situation and modify the correct responses for the materials-needed situation, such that Michelle only needs to notify her supervisor of the problem. Bella also needs to modify the correct responses for the supervisor-available situation due to the telehealth format of the assessment. In particular, returning to the workroom is not a relevant response, so Bella will record whether Michelle works on other available tasks and then calls out for the supervisor again.

Based on additional information obtained from Michelle's mother, Bella also decides to collect data on complaints or protests and inappropriate questions, along with confirming statements. She will use the ***opportunity-based format*** of the ***Additional Behaviors Data Collection Sheet*** to collect data on confirming statements and the ***frequency-based format*** of this sheet to collect data on the inappropriate behaviors. To successfully track these behaviors, Bella establishes the following definitions:

- Confirming Statements – Saying "OK," "I got it," "Will do," or similar expressions to indicate understanding when given instructions.
- Complaints/Protests – Expressing displeasure or stating that she will not follow instructions.
- Inappropriate Conversation – Asking nonwork-related questions of a personal nature or conveying information of a personal nature.

Bella will record whether or not Michelle makes a confirming statement whenever she delivers a task instruction and will record a hash mark whenever Michelle engages in complaints, protests, or inappropriate conversation during each appointment. She has selected the frequency-based format for these inappropriate behaviors because they can occur at any time during the assessment. Further, because Bella does not expect them to occur at very high levels, they likely would be easy to document throughout each appointment. Figure 7.12 shows her Additional Behaviors Data Collection Sheet.

Step 8: Conduct the VSSA

Bella now has everything that she needs to conduct the VSSA; however, before she begins, she must decide how she will respond to Michelle's inappropriate behaviors, as discussed in Chapter 4. During the initial information gathering, Michelle's mother reported that she typically ignores Michelle's complaints and protests. However, she was not sure how other people in Michelle's life typically responds to the behavior. Her mother also reported that people generally either answer Michelle's inappropriate questions or ignore them. Based on this information, Bella decides to ignore Michelle's complaints and protests and to either answer or not answer any inappropriate questions depending on the nature of the question.

Opportunity-Based Recording

Scoring: (+) correct; (-) incorrect

Date													# correct	# of opp.	%
Opportunities or Session #															
Confirming Statements															

Frequency Recording

Scoring: (/) for each occurrence of the behavior

Date/Session #/Time (min)			Total #	Total min	Rate (#/min)
Complaints/Protests					
Rate (#/min):					
Inappropriate Conversation					
Rate (#/min):					

Figure 7.12 Bell's Additional Behaviors Data Collection Sheet for Michelle's VSSA.

She follows her VSSA plan and completes it in three appointments. Occasionally, Bella and Michelle had some connectivity issues, but they resulted in very minimal disruption to the assessment. On several occasions, Michelle sought her mother's assistance with tasks and materials. However, each time, her mother simply directed her to work with Bella.

Step 9: Summarize and Interpret the VSSA

Once Bella completes the VSSA, she gathers all of the data sheets to summarize the observations and completes the calculations described in Chapter 6. She begins with the *Arranged Situations Data Sheet*. As she is reviewing the sheet, Bella notices a clear difference in Michelle's response to vague instructions versus tasks not in her repertoire. Thus, she summarizes and separates the data for these two situations. Her calculations for all situations on this data sheet are shown in Table 7.17.

Next, Bella summarizes the data on confirming statements, complaints/protests, and inappropriate conversation from the *Additional Behaviors Data Collection Sheets*. She found that Michelle never made any confirming statements, engaged in 6 complaints and protests, and asked Bella one inappropriate question ("Have you ever had a miscarriage?") during the course of the three VSSA appointments.

Step 10: Select Targets for Instruction

After transferring the data from her summaries to the *VSSA Results Report Form,* a portion of which is shown in Figure 7.13, Bella meets

Table 7.17 Summary of Michelle's performance during the arranged situations of the VSSA

Arranged Situations, Responses, & Percentage of Opportunities With Correct Responses

Task Interrupted • Completes new task = 100% • Returns to initial task = 0%	Task Completed • Seeks supervisor = 100% • Requests help = 100%
Materials Needed • Seeks assistance = 100% • Requests help = 100%	Feedback Provided • Acknowledges feedback = 0% • Asks for clear feedback = 100% • Confirms understanding = 0% • Corrects mistake = 100%
Vague Instructions • Seeks assistance = 0% • Requests help = 0%	Multiple Tasks • Correct transitions = 100%
Task Not in Repertoire • Seeks assistance = 100% • Requests help = 100%	Supervisor Unavailable • Works on other tasks = 0% • Calls out again = 0%

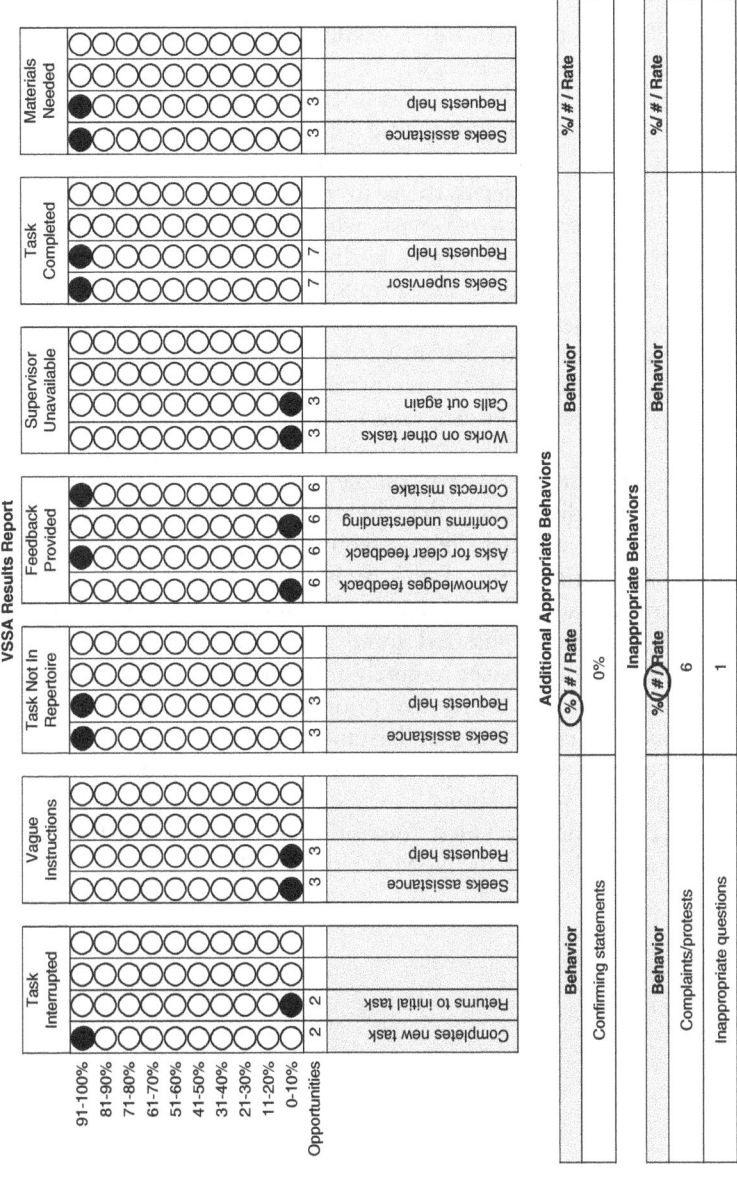

Figure 7.13 A portion of Michelle's completed VSSA Results Report Form.

with Michelle, her mother, and Michelle's vocational counselor to review the results and discuss whether Michelle would benefit from intervention prior to receiving job placement services. As they reviewed the results, they considered Michelle's preferred job settings and responsibilities and the likely social and problem-solving skills needed to successfully maintain employment in those settings.

Bella pointed to Michelle's numerous strengths, such as asking for help when she needed materials, completed her work, or was assigned a task that was not in her repertoire. She transitioned across multiple tasks independently and completed them in the instructed order, and she immediately switched to a new task when Bella asked her to do so. Although she never acknowledged feedback or confirmed her understanding of the instructions, she always asked for clear feedback and corrected her mistakes.

Bella then discussed potential areas for improvement, including asking for clarification when given vague instructions about a new task and working on other tasks when her supervisor was unavailable to assist her. Bella also noted that Michelle occasionally complained or protested when given a task; however, she always completed her work.

Next, the group discussed which skills and behaviors to prioritize for intervention in light of Michelle's preference to work in a small retail or department store and some of the problematic behaviors that might interfere with successful employment (complaints, protests, inappropriate questions). Bella also emphasized some of the practical constraints of providing intervention services remotely rather than in person. Based on these considerations, they decided to prioritize asking for help with new tasks if needed and confirming understanding of task instructions. This latter skill was selected as a replacement behavior for complaints and protests when given unstructions.

Chapter 12 provides a detailed description of the steps that Bella takes to develop and implement the VSSI for these skills.

8 Setting up the VSSI Protocol

Introducing the VSSI

Research has overwhelmingly demonstrated the effectiveness of behavior-analytic interventions for teaching new skills to learners with neurodevelopmental disabilities. At the same time, studies have shown that intervention is best when it is individualized to the learner. Rather than taking a "one size fits all approach," intervention should be tailored to the needs and responsiveness of the learner. While some learners may benefit from more intensive training and support, others may respond very well to relatively simple, time-efficient interventions. With this in mind, the VSSI protocol takes a response-to-intervention approach for identifying effective, individualized interventions for learners. Among the approaches included in the VSSI protocol are verbal and written instructions, modeling, feedback, prompts, and reinforcement. To conduct the VSSI, the instructor starts with the least intensive intervention that is likely to be effective for the learner and then progresses to more intensive interventions until the learner meets their goals.

Like the VSSA, the VSSI is conducted in authentic work situations and focuses on the measurement and monitoring of performance. Unlike the VSSA, the VSSI includes specific goals and criteria for success. The VSSI protocol also distinguishes among several separate but important aspects of training, including the initial acquisition of the target behavior, maintenance of the learner's performance over time, and generalization of the learner's behavior across different contexts, settings, and tasks. This chapter describes the steps needed to prepare for the VSSI.

Preparing for the VSSI

Chapter 6 described how the instructor should select skills or behaviors for intervention based on the results of the VSSA. Once the instructor has identified the learner's targets for intervention, the next step is to identify acquisition goals, tasks, and the relevant arranged situations to include in the VSSI.

DOI: 10.4324/9781003311935-8

Setting Goals

Establishing objective, measurable performance criteria for the learner is essential for evaluating the learner's progress, modifying the intervention as needed, and identifying when the learner has met their goals during the VSSI. The instructor should consider a variety of factors when selecting these criteria. These factors include the likely performance level needed to be successful on the job and the expectations of the learner's current and potential future employers. For example, an employee who always asks for help when needed is more likely to be successful on the job compared to an employee who asks for help just 50% of the time. On the other hand, employees probably do not need to make confirming statements every time they receive instructions or always orient towards others when speaking. Nonetheless, the instructor might want to set more stringent goals related to the initial acquisition of targeted behaviors than they would set for the maintenance of performance over time. Research suggests that requiring learners to perform at relatively high levels prior to terminating the initial stage of intervention (i.e., prior to intervention fading) can increase the likelihood that performance will maintain.

The instructor also should consult with the learner when establishing their goals. It is an important part of the collaborative process, which is intended to promote the learner's autonomy and help gain "buy in" from the learner. When doing so, the instructor should explain the rationale behind the recommended goals and provide opportunities for the learner to modify these goals based on their own preferences and aspirations.

Essential Elements of Goals

Goals for initial intervention should include the following elements: (a) the definition of a correct response (i.e., the criteria for considering a response as "correct"), (b) the desired level of performance (e.g., correct responses on 100% of opportunities; remaining on task for at least 80% of intervals), and (c) the consecutive number of opportunities, sessions, or workdays that the learner must meet the desired level of performance (e.g., across three work sessions, across 10 opportunities). In many cases, the definition of a correct response will be identical or similar to that employed during the VSSA. The instructor might make some modifications to the definition when preparing for the VSSI if further information from employers or the preferences of the learner, their caregivers, or other stakeholders suggest a different response may be more beneficial.

The following are some example goals for a sample of potential targets from the VSSA.

- Target: Responding to Corrective Feedback

  Goal: When Jerry is given corrective feedback, he will acknowledge the feedback by saying, "thank you," "I appreciate the feedback," or "I'm sorry about that" and then immediately correct his mistake on 100% of opportunities across three workdays.

- Target: Responding Appropriately When Supervisor is Unavailable

  Goal: When Shayla needs assistance to complete her work and discovers that her supervisor is unavailable, she will complete other work or ask a coworker for assistance on 100% of six consecutive opportunities.

- Target: On-Task Behavior

  Goal: Dayden will remain on-task for at least 80% of 5-minute intervals across five consecutive work sessions.

- Target: Confirming Understanding

  Goal: When assigned a new task, Octavia will confirm understanding of the task instructions by repeating the instructions and letting her supervisor know that she will complete it on at least 80% of 15 opportunities.

The case examples presented at the end of this chapter and in Chapter 12 provide additional exemplars of potential goals. To reiterate, these goals describe the criteria for determining when the learner has "mastered" the target. At that point, the instructor should initiate plans for fading the intervention and evaluating both maintenance and generalization of performance. The instructor should develop separate goals for both maintenance and generalization. These steps will be covered in Chapter 11.

Intermediate Goals

It should be noted that the learner's typical level of performance prior to intervention (i.e., "baseline") might suggest that the desired goals could take a relatively long time to achieve. For example, suppose a learner typically remains on task for less than 10% of the time, and the goal is to increase this to at least 80%. In this case, the instructor might set an intermediate, or short-term, goal that is more realistic for the learner to achieve during the VSSI. For example, the instructor could establish a goal to remain on task at least 50% of the time during the VSSI, with a plan to eventually set the goal to 80% once the learner has achieved the intermediate goal. Further information about how to obtain baseline levels of performance appears later in this chapter.

Intervention-Change Criteria

As discussed further in Chapter 9, the response-to-intervention approach of the VSSI also requires the instructor to establish criteria for modifying the intervention (i.e., progressing to more intensive training) in the event that the learner does not make adequate progress. Ideally, the "intervention-change criteria" ensures that the learner has sufficient time to make progress under the current intervention but also does not unduly prolong the VSSI by delaying needed changes to the intervention. The criteria should specify the amount of time, opportunities, or sessions by which the learner should demonstrate some progress. The required amount of progress could range from *any* increase in performance beyond the level observed in the VSSA to the attainment of the goal for acquisition. For example, the criteria could state that the instructor will modify the intervention if the learner's performance remains below a certain level (e.g., 50% of opportunities) for three consecutive work sessions or if the learner's performance does not reach the mastery criterion within five work sessions. The instructor will need to consider the learner's prior rate of progress when learning new skills and the characteristics of the intervention when selecting the intervention-change criteria. Guidelines and considerations for the selection of these criteria will be discussed in more detail in Chapter 9.

Selecting the Situations

Like the VSSA, the instructor will need to identify the situations during which it would be important for the learner to exhibit the target behaviors. The instructor will conduct the VSSI within the context of these situations. They likely will be the same situations arranged for those targets in the VSSA. For some skills, however, it will be important to vary the situation throughout the VSSI, as this will help promote generalization. For example, suppose the target is to respond appropriately when the supervisor is unavailable. It would be helpful to vary the reasons that the learner requires the supervisor's assistance during the VSSI (e.g., they have completed all of their work and don't know what to do next; they have run out of materials). As another example, suppose that the target is to relay information to others. When conducting the VSSI, the instructor might vary the recipient of the information, the location of the recipient, and the type of information to relay. This strategy will be discussed in greater detail in Chapter 11.

Selecting the Tasks

The instructor also will need to select the tasks to assign during the VSSI. It is recommended that the instructor revisit the guidelines and considerations for selecting tasks discussed in Chapter 4. In addition, the instructor should consider the potential importance of ensuring that the learner practices the targeted skills while working on a wide variety of tasks, another strategy to help promote generalization, as discussed in more detail in Chapter 11. Selecting different tasks will be particularly important when targeting responses that occur during the vague-instructions and task-not-in-repertoire situations. The assigned task must be unfamiliar to the learner each time the instructor arranges one of these situations in the VSSI. The instructor may find it challenging to procure a sufficient number of unfamiliar tasks, particularly if the learner requires a substantial number of VSSI sessions to acquire the targeted response(s). The list of potential tasks included in Appendix A may be useful in this situation.

Selecting the Interventions

The VSSI protocol includes a number of potential interventions, arranged within a recommended hierarchy, that can be evaluated for individual learners using a response-to-intervention approach. A number of factors will determine whether an instructor includes some or all of these potential interventions in the VSSI. The interventions selected for the VSSI and elements of the interventions should be individualized to the learner. Detailed descriptions of the interventions, along with guidelines for selecting, individualizing, and implementing them, will be discussed in Chapter 9.

Developing the Intervention Plan

Like the VSSA, it can be helpful to create a plan when preparing to conduct the VSSI. The plan should include the targeted behaviors, tasks, arranged situation(s), and intervention(s) to be implemented in each intervention session. Unlike the VSSA plans described in Chapters 4 and 7, the entirety of the VSSI plan cannot be predetermined. Plans for some of the VSSI sessions are dependent on the outcomes of prior sessions. As such, instructors should consider the VSSI plan to be a working document, with just a small number of sessions specified in advance and with the flexibility to adjust plans midstream. As discussed in Chapter 10, the instructor will collect data and monitor performance throughout the VSSI to permit immediate, data-based decisions that will increase the likelihood of successful outcomes. Nonetheless, the instructor will find it helpful to begin with a general, overall plan that includes the items noted above. Example plans appear at the end of this chapter and in Chapter 12.

One important aspect to consider is the number of different skills that the instructor will target at a time. Suppose, for example, that an instructor decides to target asking for help with materials, responding appropriately to feedback, and remaining on task for extended periods of time. To do so, the instructor plans to arrange for the learner to run out of materials, to receive corrective feedback, and to complete lengthy assigned tasks during work sessions. Should the instructor implement the VSSI for all three skills simultaneously? Some learners will find it challenging to work on more than one new skill at a time. For those learners, the instructor should start with one skill (e.g., asking for help with materials) until the learner has met the mastery criteria specified in their goal. Only then should the instructor introduce the intervention for a second skill (e.g., responding appropriately to feedback). While doing so, the instructor should ensure that the learner maintains their performance for the first skill. Indeed, the instructor might be even more successful if they begin to fade the intervention for the first skill before they introduce the intervention for the next one. Strategies for fading interventions to promote maintenance will be discussed further in Chapter 11.

Some learners may struggle to acquire skills that contain multiple responses. For example, responding appropriately to corrective feedback might include acknowledging the feedback, asking for clear feedback (if needed), confirming understanding of the feedback, and correcting the mistake. Although some learners may have no difficulty working on all of these component responses simultaneously, the instructor may need to focus on just one response (e.g., acknowledging the feedback) before targeting the additional responses. Many learners benefit by breaking down skills into their component responses (as illustrated for responding to feedback) and teaching one response at a time. That is, the instructor might create a task analysis of the skill and teach it as a logical sequence of component responses via chaining procedures, as described in Chapter 3. For example, the instructor might start by teaching the learner to say, "thank you for checking my work," when given corrective feedback. Once the learner has mastered this response, the instructor might teach the learner to ask for clear feedback (if needed) immediately after acknowledging the response. As the learner acquires each new response in the sequence or chain, the instructor introduces teaching for the next response. Illustrations of this approach will be presented as part of the case examples at the end of this chapter and Chapter 12.

In summary, creating the initial VSSI plan requires the instructor to determine what to target first, what intervention plans to try, and the criteria for continuing or removing one, etc. Throughout the VSSI, the instructor will continue to monitor progress by assigning tasks and arranging the relevant situations as described for the VSSA.

Conducting Baseline

The learner's performance prior to the VSSI offers a good frame of reference for identifying and evaluating improvements in their behavior once they begin to receive the intervention. This baseline level of performance can be drawn from the VSSA. If a noteworthy amount of time has passed since the completion of the VSSA, the instructor might consider repeating relevant portions of the assessment to determine whether the learner's performance has changed in the interim. The instructor also might consider collecting additional assessment data on the targeted skills if they noticed quite a bit of variability during the initial VSSA or have concerns that they did not obtain an adequate sample of their performance.

Case Example

Let's now return to the case example, John. At this point, Charise has completed her analysis of John's VSSA and selected his targets. As described in Chapter 6, she selected the following targets:

- Makes confirming statement when given a new task or feedback
- Acknowledges feedback
- Seeks assistance when given an unknown task or difficult deadline
- Makes appropriate help statement when given an unknown task or difficult deadline
- Begins additional tasks when supervisor is unavailable

Training Goals

Charise's first step in preparing for John's VSSI is to establish his acquisition goals, or the criteria by which she will determine if he has mastered the targeted skills. (His goals for maintenance and generalization will be presented in Chapter 11). In collaboration with John, she makes the following decisions. Charise recognizes and explains to John that the typical worker is unlikely to make a confirming statement every time they are given a new task or feedback. However, she wants to ensure that this behavior is strong in John's repertoire before she terminates the training. Thus, she recommends a criterion of 100% correct responses across six consecutive opportunities, with at least three occurring when he receives a new task and at least three occurring when he receives corrective feedback. Charise also explains to John that the remaining behaviors are critical to success on the job and should be performed at very high levels. In collaboration with John, she sets the acquisition goals shown in Table 8.1.

Selecting the Situations and Tasks

The next step is for Charise to consider the situations that she should include in the VSSI. The situations in Table 8.2 are directly relevant to John's targeted behaviors.

Overall, Charise will need to arrange five situations (new task instructions, corrective feedback, vague instructions, time pressure, and supervisor unavailable) while targeting his skills. Some of these situations

Table 8.1 John's acquisition goals

Behaviors	Acquisition Goal
Makes confirming statement when given new tasks or feedback	100% across 6 opportunities, 3 per arranged situation
Acknowledges feedback	100% across 3 opportunities
Seeks assistance when given unknown tasks or difficult deadlines	100% across 6 opportunities, 3 per arranged situation
Makes appropriate help statement when given unknown tasks or difficult deadlines	100% across 6 opportunities, 3 per arranged situation
Begins additional tasks when supervisor is unavailable	100% across 3 opportunities

Table 8.2 John's arranged situations

Behaviors	Arranged Situations
Makes confirming statement	New Task Instructions, Feedback Provided
Acknowledges feedback	Feedback Provided
Seeks assistance	Vague Instructions, Time Pressure
Makes appropriate help statement	Vague Instructions, Time Pressure
Begins additional tasks	Supervisor Unavailable

naturally combine. For example, she could arrange to be unavailable at times when John will need to seek assistance (when given vague instructions or time pressure). Based on her prior experiences with John, she believes he might struggle to learn all of the skills at one time. However, she thinks that he would be successful in learning two or three at a time. She notices that two of the targeted behaviors – seeks assistance and makes appropriate help statement – should occur during two different situations (vague instructions and time pressure). She decides to target those two behaviors first, along with the behavior of beginning additional tasks when the supervisor is unavailable, which she can readily arrange by being unavailable occasionally when he needs assistance. Once he has acquired those three skills, she plans to target making a confirming statement and acknowledging feedback.

Because Charise will give John vague instructions during the VSSI, she must be prepared to give him a new unfamiliar task each time she arranges this situation. With the assistance of the task list in Appendix A, Charise begins to select tasks for the VSSI, including those that she has never given John before (for the vague-instructions situation), and materials that she will need for the assigned tasks.

Table 8.3 John's initial VSSI plan

Session #	Target(s)	Situation(s)	Task(s)	Materials
1	Seeks assistance; Asks for help	Vague Instructions	Testing batteries	15 batteries; Battery tester
2	Seeks assistance; Asks for help	Vague Instructions	Making library cards	20 cards; stamp; ink
3	Seeks assistance; Asks for help	Time pressure	Sorting office supplies	20 pads; 20 pencils; 20 boxes of staples
4	Seeks assistance; Asks for help; Works on other tasks when supervisor unavailable	Vague Instructions; Supervisor Unavailable	Folding socks	15 pairs of socks
5	Seeks assistance; Asks for help	Time pressure	Pricing groceries	25 grocery items; stickers; pen
6	Seeks assistance; Asks for help; Works on other tasks when supervisor unavailable	Time pressure; Supervisor Unavailable	Shredding documents	Electric shredder; Stack of documents

Intervention Plan

Table 8.3 illustrates the beginning stages of Charise's plan. She lists the targets, situations, tasks, and materials needed for the first six sessions of the VSSI. When planning the sessions, Charise randomly arranges the order of the different situations to create a more authentic work environment. For example, in a typical work setting, John is unlikely to experience vague instructions every other assigned work task. Charise could even omit the arranged situations during some work sessions, so that John experiences some "problem-free" assignments.

The final component that Charise still needs to include in her plan is the intervention that she will implement in each session. Chapter 9 will describe the interventions in greater detail and return to this case example.

9 Conducting the VSSI

Chapter 8 outlined the initial steps that an instructor should take when preparing to implement the VSSI. This included establishing goals, identifying relevant situations, selecting the tasks and materials, and creating the VSSI plan. The final step in preparing for the VSSI is to select the interventions and the hierarchical arrangement for their implementation. The instructor then implements the VSSI as planned and makes data-based decisions to determine when the learner has met their initial acquisition goals. This chapter provides detailed descriptions and guidelines for implementing five potential interventions. Chapter 10 provides details about data collection and monitoring during the VSSI. Chapter 11 discusses how to maintain skills and promote generalization across settings, people, and contexts.

Interventions Overview

The interventions included in the VSSI are based on the principles of applied behavior analysis, as described in Chapter 3, and are supported by more than 60 years of research and practice. The recommended interventions are by no means exhaustive but have been selected because the instructor or work supervisor can implement them with relatively minimal preparation and materials, and they seem fairly practical for the workplace. These recommended interventions, however, vary in terms of their intensity, the amount of time required to implement them, and the potential for disruption to ongoing work routines. As such, the VSSI takes a response-to-intervention approach. It is recommended to start with the least intensive intervention that is likely to be effective and then move to more intensive components as needed. Nearly all learners will be successful with at least one intervention included in the VSSI.

The following is a brief description of each intervention. The first two interventions are implemented outside the context of work sessions, with the aim to prepare the learner to respond appropriately when the relevant situation(s) subsequently arise on the job. The remaining interventions,

DOI: 10.4324/9781003311935-9

designated with the label "in-situ," are conducted within the context of authentic work situations.

a **Spoken and written instructions:** The instructor begins by providing a concise but complete description of the expected behavior; the condition(s) under which it should occur; and simple, clear rationales for engaging in the behavior. Brief text may accompany the spoken instructions, using words and phrasing that are within the learner's reading comprehension ability.

b **Behavioral skills training (BST):** This multi-component intervention builds upon the spoken and written instructions described previously. After describing the expected behaviors, the instructor models them for the learner and then instructs the learner to practice the behaviors in brief roleplay scenarios with the instructor. The instructor provides immediate feedback for both correct and incorrect responses. These practice trials continue until the learner meets a mastery criterion, usually by engaging in the response correctly for a certain number of consecutive practice attempts.

c **In-situ feedback.** The instructor arranges relevant situations during work sessions as described in the VSSI plan or takes advantage of naturally occurring situations. The instructor then monitors the learner's behavior and provides positive or corrective feedback about their performance.

d **In-situ prompts, including spoken, visual, and technology.** The instructor provides spoken, written, or technology-delivered prompts, or "cues," to help the learner respond correctly during arranged or naturally occurring situations. Prompts may be delivered before the learner has an opportunity to respond to the relevant situation or after the learner encounters the situation and responds incorrectly. The former arrangement is designed to prevent errors before they occur, whereas the latter arrangement provides an opportunity for the learner to correct their errors.

e **In-situ reinforcement.** The instructor builds upon the feedback and prompts described previously by identifying and providing tangible reinforcement for correct responses.

Consequences for Work Completion

As described in Chapter 3, behaviors are a function of their consequences. Thus, it is important to consider what reinforcing consequences will maintain the skills targeted for intervention beyond any contrived reinforcers delivered by the instructor. The ability to complete assigned tasks successfully is the immediate natural consequence for many of the recommended social skills, such as asking for help when needed and responding appropriately to feedback. For this reason, it is crucial to ascertain whether task completion is reinforcing to the learner. For some learners, task completion itself is a conditioned reinforcer due to a prior history of receiving social or tangible reinforcers for completing tasks. Paychecks and continued employment also may reinforce successful task completion for learners who are participating in paid employment. Learners likely fall into this category if they tend to remain on task when given all necessary instructions and materials, seem eager to finish their work, and persist in responding until tasks are completed. Instructors only need to ensure that these learners acquire the targeted social skills, as these new behaviors will result in the natural consequence of successful task completion and any additional reinforcers associated with this success.

For other learners, particularly those who need to improve their on-task behavior, the instructor should identify and arrange reinforcers for task completion. Such a strategy will help ensure that the learner remains motivated to perform newly acquired job skills. Tips and guidelines for implementing this approach are provided later in this chapter under the section *in-situ reinforcement*. The instructor also may need to arrange reinforcement for other targeted behaviors that have subtle, delayed, or weak natural consequences. Examples of behaviors that likely fall into this category for some learners include making confirming statements in response to instructions and orienting toward listeners when speaking. Although these behaviors can improve social relationships on the job, this consequence may develop very gradually over time and may not be readily apparent or highly effective as a reinforcer for the learner.

Structuring the VSSI

As part of the response-to-intervention approach, the instructor will select a hierarchy of interventions to include in the VSSI from among those rec-ommended in this chapter. The instructor will begin by implementing the first intervention for the targeted response(s). The instructor will then evaluate the effects of the intervention on the learner's performance during authentic work situations based on the established goals and criteria, as described in Chapter 8. If the intervention is deemed insufficient, the instructor will proceed to the next intervention in the planned hierarchy and evaluate its effectiveness. This process will continue until the learner meets the desired goal for those response(s). If the instructor has additional behaviors to target, they can either reimplement the response-to-intervention approach or use the intervention that was shown to be effective with the prior skill(s). For example, recall that in Chapter 8, John's instructor, Charise, decided to begin his VSSI by targeting three of five behaviors identified as needing improvement: (a) seeks assistance, (b) makes appropriate help statements, and (c) begins additional tasks when the supervisor is not available. Suppose Charise determined that her first intervention, spoken and written instructions, was not sufficient to improve any of those skills.

However, John met his acquisition goals when she moved to her second intervention, BST. For the remaining two targets (makes confirming statement and acknowledges feedback), Charise may implement BST as her first intervention rather than evaluating the effects of spoken and written instructions, under the reasonable assumption that those skills are unlikely to improve with instructions alone.

Data-Based Decision Making

The VSSI plan should be considered a "working document" that is directly informed by the learner's performance. The instructor will need to establish criteria for continuing to evaluate the effects of a particular intervention in the hierarchy or moving on to the next planned intervention. As discussed in Chapter 8, this is the "intervention-change criterion." For example, in the case example at the end of this chapter, the instructor decides that she will introduce the next intervention if the learner's performance does not improve during the relevant arranged situation two times. As long as she sees improvement she will continue to evaluate his performance until he meets the acquisition criterion. Additional details about data collection, analysis, and interpretation during the VSSI will be described in Chapter 10.

Recommended Interventions for the VSSI

In this section, each intervention is described in greater detail, along with considerations for using it with learners. As noted previously, the first two interventions are implemented outside the context of work sessions, with the aim to prepare the learner to respond appropriately when the relevant situation(s) arise. They are considered less intrusive than the remaining interventions because the instructor does not need to be present while the learner is on the job or completing work tasks. This restricts implementation to circumscribed times and reduces potential disruptions to others in the work area. The instructor can meet with the learner in an office or classroom to conduct the training but preferably in the same building as the work area. This may help promote the transfer of learning from the training context to the work context. The instructor would conduct any of the remaining interventions "in-situ" during authentic work situations by arranging relevant situations (as described for the VSSA) and by taking advantage of any opportunities that arise naturally on the job site.

Spoken and Written Instructions

Some learners show immediate, substantial improvements in performance when given clear rules and expectations. For these learners, spoken and written instructions are a good place to start when initiating the VSSI. Prior observations of the learner or the input of those who know the learner can be obtained to determine whether the learner has previously modified their behavior based on instructions and rules alone. If so, it is possible (although not guaranteed) that a similar intervention will prove effective for the targeted job skills.

The instructor should provide clear, concise descriptions of the expected behaviors and the situations when it would be most helpful for the learner to perform them. The instructor can explain the importance of the behaviors by describing and comparing what would happen if the learner does and does not engage in them. Ideally, the instructor should accompany the spoken instructions with brief text, using words and phrasing that are within the learner's reading comprehension ability. Graphical illustrations and pictures could potentially substitute for the text if the learner has limited reading comprehension skills. The written instructions or illustrations provide a tangible, or permanent, product that the learner can reference later, similar to textual prompts described below. When evaluating the effects of spoken and written instructions during subsequent work sessions, the instructor should ensure that the learner has access to the written materials. For example, the instructor could permit the learner to keep the written instructions in their work area or post them in a location that is easily accessible to the learner.

The following are some examples of spoken and written instructions:

Target: Responding to Vague Feedback

(Spoken instructions) "Sometimes your supervisor may tell you that you did not complete a task correctly but you still don't understand what you did wrong or how to fix it. When this happens, you should thank them for the feedback and ask them to show you how to correct the mistake. If you don't ask them to show you how to fix your mistake, you may continue to do the work incorrectly and your supervisor may think that you are not following their instructions and will become annoyed with you. If you ask your supervisor to show you, you will be able to complete the task correctly and your supervisor will consider you to be a good worker who listens to feedback.

Corresponding written instructions are shown in Figure 9.1, and corresponding simplified written instructions with pictures are shown in Figure 9.2.

If the supervisor tells you to fix your work and you don't understand how to fix it:

1. Thank your supervisor for the feedback.
2. Ask your supervisor to show you how to fix your work.
3. Tell the supervisor you will fix the task.
4. Fix your mistakes and finish the task.

Figure 9.1 Example written instructions.

You made a mistake but don't know what to do:

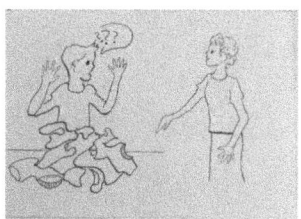

Thank supervisor   Ask supervisor how   Say you will fix it   Fix it

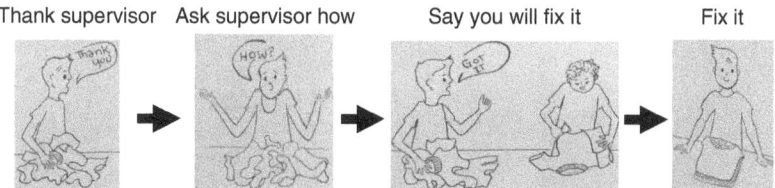

Figure 9.2 Example simplified written instructions with pictures. Drawings by Roberta Lerman. Used with permission by the artist.

Target: Responding When Task Is Interrupted

(Spoken Instructions) "Sometimes your supervisor may interrupt you when you are working on an assigned task and ask you to complete a different task first. When this happens, it usually means that the new task is more important to complete at that time. Thus, you should immediately switch to the new task, let your supervisor know when it is completed, and then return to finish the interrupted one. By doing so, your supervisor will see that you are a hard worker who listens to instructions and understands the need to get the job done. If you don't, your supervisor will think that you don't listen and that they cannot depend on you to get the job done."

Corresponding written instructions are shown in Figure 9.3, and corresponding simplified written instructions with pictures are shown in Figure 9.4

If the supervisor interrupts your work to give you a new task:
1. Finish the new task.
2. Tell the supervisor you are done with the new task.
3. Finish the first task you were working on.

Figure 9.3 Example written instructions.

If supervisor stops you and gives you new task:

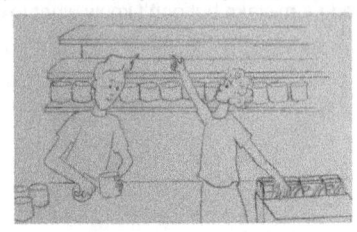

Do new task.   Tell supervisor Done   Go back to first task

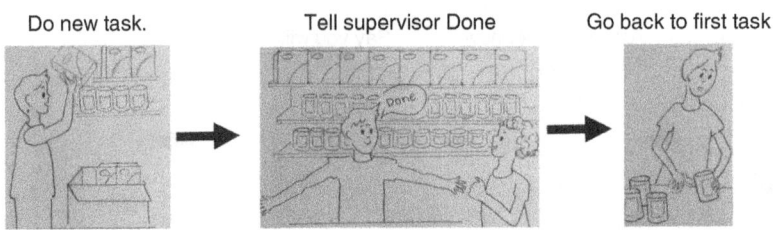

Figure 9.4 Example simplified written instructions with pictures. Drawings by Roberta Lerman. Used with permission by the artist.

It also can be helpful to pose questions to the learner to check their understanding of the information. For example, the instructor might ask the following questions after the relevant portion(s) of the spoken/written instructions or at the end of the presentation:

• Why is it important to engage in this response?
• What will happen if you don't engage in this response?
• What will happen if you do engage in this response?
• What are the steps that you should take in the situation?

Any incorrect answers would result in corrective feedback and review of the relevant instructions. The instructor also may choose to re-present all of the questions again until the learner answers them correctly.

Behavioral Skills Training (BST)

This multi-step intervention includes modeling, practice in roleplay, and feedback. BST consists of the following steps:

STEP 1: The instructor describes the expected behaviors and why they are important. Guidelines for providing these instructions are identical to those described in the prior section.

STEP 2: The instructor models the expected behavior(s) for the learner at least one time but may model multiple times if the learner would benefit from repetition. The instructor also might consider including models of both correct and incorrect instances of the behavior. The instructor can check for understanding by having the learner identify which models are correct examples and which models are incorrect examples.

STEP 3: The instructor has the learner practice the behaviors in brief roleplay scenarios with the instructor, who provides immediate feedback for both correct and incorrect responses. To set up the scenarios, the instructor will need to ask the learner to pretend that they are on a job site and then describe the scene. For example, while showing the learner some task materials, the instructor might say, "Here is a task. I want you to pretend that you don't understand how to complete it. I want you to practice what I just showed you." The instructor will then pretend to give the learner the task to complete and observe how the learner responds. The instructor will describe what the learner does correctly (e.g., "Nice job telling me that you have never done this task before!") as well as what they did incorrectly ("But you should also ask me to show you how to complete it."). The instructor should vary the task materials and situation as much as possible to help promote transfer of learning to the job site. Practice role plays continue until the learner meets a mastery criterion, usually by engaging in the response correctly for a certain number of consecutive practice attempts.

In-situ Feedback

If BST does not lead to behavior change during authentic work situations, the instructor would begin to deliver feedback to the learner about their performance during work sessions. This requires the instructor to closely monitor the learner's behavior during arranged or naturally occurring situations that are relevant to the targeted skill(s). When the learner responds correctly, the instructor provides immediate, descriptive praise (e.g., "Nicely done! You let me know when you had finished your task and asked what you could do next."). When the learner responds incorrectly, the instructor provides immediate corrective feedback by describing what the learner did incorrectly and what they should do instead (e.g., "You went to the break room when I was unavailable but you should have found other work to do.") The instructor also may provide a quick model and opportunity for practice within the context of corrective feedback.

In-situ Prompts (Spoken, Visual, and Technology-Delivered)

If in-situ feedback does not lead to improved performance, embedding prompts within authentic work situations can help the learner respond correctly at the right moment. The instructor will need to select the modality of the prompt (spoken, visual, or technology-delivered) and the timing of the prompt (before or after the learner has an opportunity to respond). When choosing the modality, the instructor should consider the types of prompts that likely would be feasible and acceptable on the job site, as well as the types of prompts that have been effective with the learner in the past. For example, some work sites may prohibit employees from using personal cell phones or other handheld devices while working, which might eliminate the possibility of technology-delivered prompts. The instructor also should consider the preferences of the learner and permit them to choose among several possible types of prompts. Most important, the learner should reliably respond correctly when they receive the selected prompt (i.e., the prompt should be effective). Finally, the instructor should consider whether the selected prompt would be easy to fade from the work environment to help promote the learner's independence. The following are commonly used prompts:

- Spoken prompts are hints or reminders about the correct response. For example, the instructor might say to the learner, "Don't forget to come find me if you run out of materials," or "Say, 'Can you show me how?'" The former prompt could be delivered either before or after the learner has encountered the relevant situation (i.e., when the learner runs out of materials). The latter prompt, which models what the learner should say to the supervisor when they don't know how to complete an assigned task, would be delivered once the learner has received vague instructions or an unfamiliar task.

- Visual prompts consist of gestures, models, text, or pictures. For example, the instructor might gesture towards the supply cabinet or search the cabinet themselves (i.e., model) when the learner runs out of materials. They might create a card printed with the instruction, "Find your supervisor when you are done with your task," or a phrase that specifies what the learner should say to the supervisor when they are finished with their work, such as "I'm done. What's next?" Instructions like the former textual prompt could be delivered either before or after the learner encounters the relevant situation. The latter textual prompt, which specifies what the learner should say to the supervisor when they have finished with their work, typically would be delivered when it is appropriate for the learner to emit the response. For this type of prompt, the instructor should consider providing multiple examples of statements to prevent rote responding. For example, the card could include the phrases, "I'm done with my work. What else can I do?" "Finished. What would you like me to do now?" and "All done. What's next"? All textual prompts should be individualized to the reading level of the learner. For learners with little to no reading skills, the instructor could substitute familiar pictures for words.

- Technology-delivered prompts can take a variety of forms but require some type of electronic or digital device, such as cell phones (e.g., automated reminders; text messages) and tablets or computers (e.g., written instructions, videos). For example, the instructor could arrange for the learner to receive an automated cell phone reminder to remain on-task every 10 minutes or send written prompts via text messages to the learner's cell phone. Although a bit more complicated to create and arrange, the instructor could download video models to a tablet, laptop, or computer that show the learner or someone else engaging in the correct response (e.g., asking the supervisor for help). The learner then could access and watch the videos when encountering the relevant situation.

The timing of the prompt typically determines whether the learner has an opportunity to make an error. If the instructor provides the prompt *before* the learner encounters the relevant situation or immediately afterwards, the learner is less likely to respond incorrectly. For example, suppose a learner's target is to work on an alternative task when the supervisor is unavailable to help with the current one. The instructor might ensure that the learner receives the prompt before they discover that the supervisor is unavailable. The instructor could do this by having a written prompt posted in the work area or by vocally stating earlier in the work session what the learner should do if their supervisor is not available to help. If the learner would benefit from a shorter latency between the prompt and the opportunity to respond, the instructor could deliver the prompt at the moment that the learner encounters this problem but before they have had an opportunity to respond. As soon as the learner discovers that the supervisor is unavailable, the instructor could send the text message, "Find other tasks to do," to the learner's cell phone, vocally state, "Find other tasks to do," or hand the learner a card with the written statement, "Find other tasks to do." This arrangement requires particular vigilance of the instructor, who must closely monitor the learner's behavior and events occurring in the environment. The advantage of these arrangements is that the learner has less opportunity to respond incorrectly during the relevant situations.

A delay between the relevant situation and the appearance of the prompt increases the likelihood that the learner will make an error. For example, instead of working on an alternative task, the learner may sit down in the break room. The instructor could respond to this error by delivering a spoken, written, or technology-delivered prompt. The learner may then engage in a correct, prompted response. However, research suggests that many learners acquire skills more quickly under "errorless" learning arrangements. A disadvantage of an errorless arrangement is that the learner may be less likely to respond independently, or without a prompt. This disadvantage highlights the importance of fading prompts, which not only ensures independence but helps promote maintenance and generalization. Prompts can be faded in a variety of ways, a topic discussed in greater detail in Chapter 11. Regardless of the type or timing of the prompts, it is recommended that instructors combine prompts with in-situ feedback as described previously.

In-situ Reinforcement

For the final recommended intervention of the VSSI, the instructor identifies and provides tangible reinforcement for correct responses to enhance the efficacy of feedback and prompts. Reinforcement can include the various types of unconditioned, conditioned, and generalized reinforcers described in Chapter 3, and requires the instructor to identify the individual preferences of the learner. Potential reinforcers include food, drink, activities (e.g., watching videos, listening to music), work breaks, preferred work tasks, and money or other types of generalized reinforcers (i.e., tokens). To identify highly preferred items, activities, and tasks, the instructor should ask the learner and their caregivers about these preferences and provide opportunities for the learner to choose among various options. Both of these methods are described in Chapter 3. The instructor also should give special consideration to any natural reinforcers for inappropriate behavior that they identified during the VSSA, such as attention from others, breaks from tasks, and access to specific tangible items. These should be particularly potent reinforcers for appropriate behavior.

The instructor will need to consider a number of other factors when selecting highly preferred items to use as reinforcement during work sessions. First, the instructor might consider whether any of the selected reinforcers would be deemed inappropriate for use at the learner's current or planned job placements. For example, some employers prohibit the consumption of food or drinks outside of scheduled break times or cannot permit workers to take extra breaks or to choose their tasks.

The instructor also should consider other potential constraints on reinforcement delivery. Reinforcement is most effective when given immediately following the desired behavior. Doing so, however, could disrupt ongoing work tasks, particularly if the reinforcer is an activity (e.g., watching a video), a break, or an opportunity to work on more preferred tasks. This may or may not be considered problematic, depending on the learner, their targets, and the job sites.

When reinforcement delivery must be delayed, the instructor should consider using generalized (conditioned) reinforcers, such as tokens or money, to help bridge the gap between the performance of the targeted behavior and access to the earned reinforcer. Generalized reinforcers permit the instructor to deliver reinforcement immediately following the desired behavior with minimal disruption to the worker's ongoing behavior (e.g., the instructor can hand the worker a poker chip or a quarter). At another time, the learner can exchange the tokens or money for highly preferred tangible or activity reinforcers (called "backup reinforcers"). Such an exchange is crucial for success because tokens derive their value from this pairing with backup reinforcers. For this reason, the instructor must carefully arrange the token system to ensure that the learner has opportunities to exchange their tokens for one or more highly preferred reinforcers at regularly scheduled times.

For example, suppose an instructor gives the learner a token whenever they have remained on task for 20 minutes and whenever they notify the supervisor that they are done with their work. The instructor might arrange for them to exchange their tokens during regularly scheduled break times. The instructor has identified soda, chips, breaks, video games, and early work release as preferred items and activities for this learner. The instructor assigns "prices" to these various backup reinforcers based on the total number of tokens the learner could possibly earn prior to each exchange and the perceived "value" of the reinforcer (more valuable reinforcers cost more). This creates the "reinforcer menu" shown in Table 9.1.

Including multiple reinforcers on the menu ensures that the learner will be interested in earning at least one of the available reinforcers during each exchange opportunity. Assigning different price points to the

Table 9.1 Example reinforcer menu for token economy

Reinforcer Menu	
Item	Price
One can of soda	3 tokens
One bag of chips	3 tokens
Extra 5 min of break	5 tokens
Leave work 5 min early	5 tokens
5 min of video gaming	6 tokens
Leave work 15 min early	10 tokens
15 min of video gaming	10 tokens

Table 9.2 Common mistakes when using reinforcement

Common Mistakes When Using Reinforcement
Offering the same reinforcers over and over.
Using reinforcers that are not powerful.
Conducting a preference assessment once and never again.
Waiting too long to give reinforcement for the desired response.
Eliminating reinforcers completely.

reinforcers increases the likelihood that the learner can purchase at least one reinforcer even if they don't earn all of the possible tokens prior to the exchange. Furthermore, the learner may be more motivated to earn as many tokens as possible by assigning the highest prices to the most valuable reinforcers.

Some common mistakes that people make when arranging reinforcement are listed in Table 9.2. Avoiding these mistakes may help ensure that in-situ reinforcement is highly effective for learners.

Although reinforcement should not be completely eliminated for behaviors that are desirable to maintain, the use of in-situ reinforcement requires a plan for fading reinforcement over time to ensure successful maintenance and generalization of the learner's performance. Strategies for reinforcement fading will be described in Chapter 11.

Case Example

In Chapter 8, instructor Charise had started to draft John's initial VSSI plan by determining which behaviors to target first, the order in which she would introduce interventions for his selected targets, the situations she would arrange, and the tasks that she would assign John. Her final step is to select the hierarchy of interventions to include in the VSSI. Charise begins by considering whether to evaluate spoken and written instructions alone. John has moderate receptive language skills and

Table 9.3 John's initial VSSI plan

Session #	Target(s)	Intervention	Situation
	John's VSSI Plan		
1	Seeks assistance; Asks for help	Written/Spoken Instructions	Vague Instructions
2	Seeks assistance; Asks for help	Written/Spoken Instructions (if needed)	Vague Instructions
3	Seeks assistance; Asks for help	Written/Spoken Instructions	Time Pressure
4	Seeks assistance; Asks for help;	BST (if needed)	Vague Instructions
	Works on other tasks when supervisor unavailable	Written/Spoken Instructions	Supervisor Unavailable
5	Seeks assistance; Asks for help	Written/Spoken Instructions (if needed)	Time Pressure
6	Seeks assistance; Asks for help;	BST (if needed)	Time Pressure
	Works on other tasks when supervisor unavailable	Written/Spoken Instructions (if needed)	Supervisor Unavailable

reads on a 6th-grade level. Charise has observed John complying with rules and instructions in the past. For these reasons, she feels that spoken and written instructions might be a viable intervention for John and selects them as the first intervention in the VSSI hierarchy. If this intervention is not successful, Charise will implement BST, followed by in-situ feedback, in-situ prompts (via cell text messaging), and in-situ reinforcement, as needed. After selecting the interventions, Charise completes the initial VSSI plan, which outlines just the first six work sessions.

As shown in Table 9.3, she plans to begin by giving John spoken and written instructions for the first two targeted behaviors (seeks assistance and asks for help), which she will target within the vague-instructions and time-pressure situations. Charise has decided that she will attempt instructions at least twice with each relevant arranged situation before moving to the next intervention if needed. Thus, if John does not respond correctly during the first work session, Charise will repeat the written and spoken instructions before she sets up the next work session in the day plan. She may or may not conduct the subsequent sessions as planned, depending on the outcomes.

Before the first work session, Charise meets with John in her office to describe how to seek assistance and ask for help when he is given task instructions that he does not understand. Charise clarifies for John what it means to get unclear instructions and describes both examples and nonexamples of this situation. She then states what John should do and why it is important to do so, making sure to use language within his comprehension. For example, she says the following:

> *Today, we are going to discuss what to do if you do not know how to do a new task. The supervisor may sometimes give you confusing instructions or a task that you have never done before. This may be a task that you have done before, but you have never done this task at your current job. For example, let's say I used to work at a department store and my supervisor there showed me how to fold clothes. I am now working at Goodwill. On my first day, the supervisor at Goodwill tells me to fold clothes but does not show or tell me how to do it. I should find my supervisor and say, "How would like me to fold the clothes?" This is important so that I can be sure to fold them correctly and not have to do them all over again. So, when you are given a new task and your supervisor does not completely show or tell you how to do it, you should find your supervisor and ask them to show or tell you how to do the task correctly. You should not just try to do the task the way that you have before and hope that it is right.*

Charise supplements this spoken description with the written statements in Figure 9.5.

If your supervisor gives you a new task but does not show you how to do it:

  1. Go to your supervisor.
  2. Ask your supervisor to show you how to do your work.

Figure 9.5 Written instructions for John.

Charise asks John questions to test for understanding and, after noting that his answers suggested that he understands the instructions, she then describes how to seek assistance and ask for help when his supervisor tells him that he must complete the work quickly (time pressure). For example, she says the following:

> *Now, we are going to discuss another situation that requires you to find your supervisor and ask for help. In this situation, your supervisor gives you a task and tells you that you must do it quickly. However, you don't think that you can do it that fast. Sometimes, a job needs to be done right away or it could be bad for the company. Your supervisor may not know that you can't do the job that fast and that you need help. So, when this happens, you should find your supervisor and say, "I can't do this fast enough. Can someone help me?" You can't get help if you don't ask. If the work is not finished quickly, it could hurt the company or your co-workers. If you get help, the work will get done when it is supposed to.*

Charise supplements this spoken description with the written statements in Figure 9.6

After John confirms that he understands the instructions, Charise then describes what John should do if his supervisor is not available when he seeks help. She provides rationales, an example and nonexample, and supplemental written instructions. Now that she has given John the instructions for the first three targeted behaviors, Charise places the written instructions in John's work area and tells John that it is time to go to work. She then follows her VSSI plan for the first several work sessions, as shown in Table 9.4.

John does not seek assistance from or ask Charise for help when she asks him to test batteries (first work session), so Charise reviews the instructions

If your supervisor asks you to complete a task quickly but you can't do it that fast:

  1. Go to your supervisor.
  2. Explain the problem.
  3. Ask if someone can help you.

Figure 9.6 Written instructions for John.

Table 9.4 First three sessions of John's VSSI plan

Session #	Target(s)	Intervention	Situation(s)	Task(s)	Materials
1	Seeks assistance; Asks for help	Written/Spoken Instructions	Vague Instructions	Test batteries	15 batteries; Battery tester
2	Seeks assistance; Asks for help	Written/Spoken Instructions	Vague Instructions	Make library cards	20 cards; stamp
3	Seeks sssistance; Asks for help	Written/Spoken Instructions	Time Pressure	Sort office supplies	20 pads; 20 pencils; 20 boxes of staples

with John before the second work session during which she gives him vague instructions for a library card-making task. However, John again does not respond correctly. When she arranges the time-pressure situation in the third session, Charise is delighted when John immediately tells her that he can't sort the office supplies quickly enough and asks for help. For the fourth work session, Charise had planned to give him vague instructions. Because John did not ask for help when he encountered vague instructions during the first two work sessions, Charise introduces BST during the fourth work session.

Charise selects some work materials and meets with John in her office. She describes and models the correct responses and asks John to practice while giving him various different types of vague instructions and work materials. She provides both positive and corrective feedback as he practices seeking her assistance and asking for help. Once John has responded correctly three times, Charise concludes the training.

When John returns to work, Charis gives him the sock folding task as shown in Table 9.5 for the fourth work session; however, she revises her original plan by removing the supervisor unavailable situation and its associated target from this session. She wants to be sure he immediately encounters the natural consequence of seeking the supervisor and asking for help if indeed he attempts to do so during this first session after BST. In fact, John responds correctly during the fourth work session, so Charise continues the VSSI as shown in Table 9.5, again evaluating his performance during the time-pressure situation. She also arranges the supervisor-unavailable situation so that she can evaluate the effects of written and spoken instructions on the associated target (i.e., working on other tasks).

Charise is delighted when John continues to ask for help correctly during the time-pressure situation; he also works on other tasks when Charise is unavailable (she pretends to be speaking to someone on the phone). In the sixth session, he again responds correctly when given vague instructions and when he discovers that Charise is not immediately available to assist him (she goes into the restroom). When she returns to his work area, he asks her how to complete the shredding task.

Table 9.5 Sessions four through six of John's VSSI plan

Session #	Target(s)	Intervention	Situation(s)	Task(s)	Materials
4	Seeks assistance; Asks for help	BST	Vague Instructions	Fold socks	15 pairs of socks
5	Seeks assistance; Asks for help; Works on other tasks when supervisor unavailable	Written/Spoken Instructions	Time Pressure; Supervisor Unavailable	Price groceries	25 grocery items; stickers; pen
6	Seeks assistance; Asks for help; Works on other tasks when supervisor unavailable		Vague Instructions; Supervisor Unavailable	Shred documents	Electric shredder; Stack of documents

In light of John's consistent performance with his first three targets, Charise decides to introduce interventions for his two remaining targets, making confirming statements and acknowledging feedback. Confirming statements is a target associated with two different situations (i.e., opportunities) – when John's supervisor gives him feedback and when John's supervisor gives him clear instructions to complete a new task. She drafts the next four sessions of his VSSI plan to include these targets, shown in Table 9.6, while still occasionally evaluating his other

Table 9.6 Sessions seven through ten of John's VSSI plan

Session #	Target(s)	Intervention	Situation(s)	Task(s)	Materials
7	Confirms understanding	Written/Spoken Instructions	Clear Instructions	Price groceries	25 grocery items; stickers; pen
8	Confirms understanding; Works on other tasks when supervisor unavailable	Written/Spoken Instructions (if needed)	Clear Instructions; Supervisor Unavailable	Stock shelves	25 grocery items; four-drawer stack
9	Seeks assistance; Asks for help; Acknowledges feedback; Confirms understanding	Written/Spoken Instructions	Vague Instructions; Feedback Provided	Fold shirts	30 shirts
10	Confirms understanding; Works on other tasks when supervisor unavailable	BST (if needed)	Clear Instructions; Supervisor Unavailable	Shred	Shredder; Stack of documents

targets to determine when he meets the acquisition criteria established in Chapter 8.

Immediately prior to the seventh session, she meets with John to go over written and spoken instructions about confirming his understanding when he gets a new task. Immediately prior to the ninth session, Charise provides written and spoken instructions about how to acknowledge his supervisor's feedback when she tells him that he has made a mistake and how to confirm that he will fix his work. As shown in the upcoming Chapter 10, John ultimately acquired all of his targets with spoken and written instructions with the exception of seeking assistance and asking for help when given vague instructions and confirming his understanding of new task instructions. For these targets, BST was highly effective for John.

10 Monitoring and Interpreting VSSI Outcomes

As discussed in Chapter 9, conducting the VSSI is a highly dynamic process that requires ongoing monitoring and evaluation of performance. Decisions about when to target skills and how to target them in each VSSI session are based strictly on performance data and the associated criteria that guide those decisions. This chapter provides details about how to summarize and display data so that instructors can readily track progress and make data-based decisions throughout the VSSI.

Collecting and Summarizing Data

Baseline

As noted in Chapter 9, data on a learner's performance *prior* to intervention, called baseline data, offer a good frame of reference for identifying and evaluating changes in the learner's skills during the VSSI. This baseline level of performance can be drawn from the VSSA and/or by repeating relevant portions of the assessment before starting the VSSI. The latter is recommended if a substantial amount of time has passed since the VSSA was completed, if the learner's behavior was quite variable during the VSSA, or if the instructor did not obtain at least three opportunities to observe the learner's performance under the relevant situation(s) during the VSSA. Certainly, the data displayed in the *VSSA Results Report Form* can serve as the learner's baseline performance. However, as discussed in the next section and later in the chapter, the instructor should summarize and inspect data from individual sessions or observations when gathering data on baseline levels of performance before introducing interventions for the VSSI.

Intervention

Data on the learner's performance should be collected during every work session. A modified version of the *Arranged Situations Data Sheet* and the *Additional Behaviors Data Sheets* from the VSSA can be used

DOI: 10.4324/9781003311935-10

during the planned VSSI sessions. However, instead of using a single data sheet to collect data across multiple work sessions, observations, or work shifts as described in Chapter 5, the instructor should collect and summarize data on a session-by-session (or observation-by-observation) basis. The following sections describe how to collect and summarize data using these sheets during the VSSI. Additional examples of collecting data via these data sheets are provided with the case example at the end of this chapter, along with those in Chapter 12.

The *VSSI Arranged Situations Template Data Sheet*, provided in Appendix B, will be helpful when collecting data during the VSSI. When collecting and summarizing data with this sheet, the instructor has the option to collapse across multiple targeted responses within the same opportunity or to examine data for each individual response separately. For example, possible learner responses when they receive corrective feedback include (a) acknowledging the feedback, (b) asking for clearer feedback if needed, (c) confirming the feedback, and (d) correcting the mistake. The instructor could determine the percentage of responses (a)–(d) that the learner completed correctly each time that they receive feedback. Figure 10.1 illustrates this approach using the *VSSI Arranged Situations Template Data Sheet.* The data collector has recorded "+" for each correct response and "–" for each incorrect one (along with an "N" if the learner had no opportunity to emit the response) in each session. Then, for each session, the data collector has divided the total number of correct responses by the total number of possible responses, multiplied the result by 100 to convert it to a percentage, and entered this value in the bottom row of each column.

Alternatively, the instructor could monitor the learner's progress for each targeted response by using a "yes"/"no" format when graphing the data, as described later in this chapter. By doing so, the instructor can more readily determine if the learner is having difficulty with certain responses. For example, as illustrated in Figure 10.1, the learner may consistently ask for clear feedback when needed and correct their mistakes but fail to acknowledge or confirm the supervisor's feedback. Examining only the summary data on the overall percentage of correct responses (displayed in the last row) shows that the learner was performing some of the responses incorrectly, but it does not reveal which response(s) the learner was struggling to acquire.

Additional Behaviors Data Sheets. When collecting and summarizing the data via these data sheets, the instructor will have all of the format options described for the VSSA in Chapter 5. This includes the opportunity-based, interval-based, and frequency- or rate-based formats. However, as noted previously, the instructor should summarize the data on a session-by-session (or observation-by-observation) basis, or at a maximum, collapse across small groups of sessions or observations (e.g., daily sessions) for the purpose of monitoring performance over time.

Situation: Feedback Provided

Date	3/5	3/5	3/8	3/9								
Session #	1	2	3	4								
Acknowledge feedback	-	-	-	-								
Ask for clearer feedback if needed	N	+	+	+								
Confirm the feedback	-	-	-	-								
Correct the mistake	+	+	+	+								
Percentage (correct/total):	33%	50%	50%	50%								

Figure 10.1 Illustrative data using the VSSI Arranged Situations Template Data Sheet.

Examples of collecting and summarizing data in this manner are provided in the next section on graphing and with the case examples at the end of this chapter and in Chapter 12.

Graphing Data

Graphical displays of the summarized data are highly recommended for monitoring performance during the VSSI and for sharing the results with the learner and other stakeholders. Graphs provide an immediate visual representation of the quantitative data that are collected on the various data sheets. Line graphs that show the learner's performance during each work session or opportunity to respond are ideal for this purpose. Plotting both baseline and intervention data on the same line graphs will enable the viewer to immediately detect changes in performance and determine when the learner has met the acquisition criteria. This section provides an overview and description of recommended graphical displays. Detailed instructions on how best to graph data collected during the VSSI will be provided later in the chapter.

A typical line graph with its essential components, including hypo-thetical data on the percentage of intervals with on-task behavior collected via the interval-based format of the ***Additional Behaviors Data Sheet***, is illustrated in Figure 10.2. Each data point shows the level of on-task behavior during each work session. Each data point aligns with its value on the horizontal axis and the session or observation number on the vertical axis.

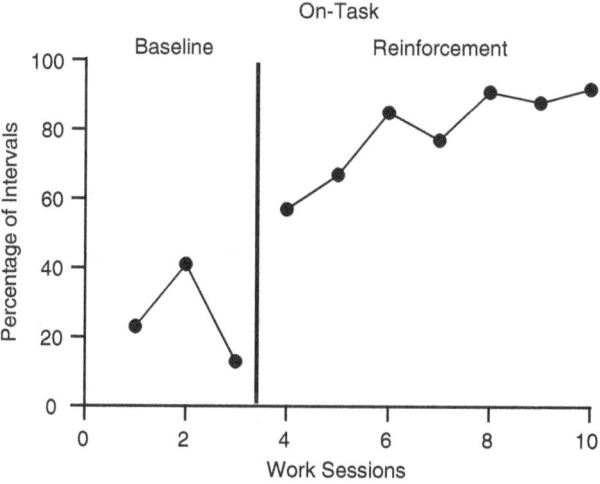

Figure 10.2 Example of line graph.

The instructor begins by plotting the baseline data, as indicated by the label "Baseline" that appears in the first panel of the graph. The instructor uses lines to connect each data point to the next one, which helps to highlight the level of performance and changes over time. Suppose the baseline data in Figure 10.2 were collected during the learner's VSSA. Instead of collapsing across all data gathered during the VSSA, as described in Chapter 6, the instructor has plotted the interval-based data for on-task behavior from the relevant work sessions. This permits a more fine-grained analysis of performance by showing session-by-session variation in the level of on-task behavior (as opposed to the overall mean level). Graphing baseline data in this manner also provides a more appropriate point of comparison for the session-by-session intervention data.

As shown in Figure 10.2, the instructor indicates the start of the intervention by entering a horizontal line on the graph, positioned immediately after the last baseline data point. The instructor then continues to graph data collected on the behavior, using lines to connect each data point to the next one. However, breaks in the line that connects the data points occur whenever a new intervention is introduced. The resulting graph provides an easy-to-read visual display of the intervention's effects on performance. The data plotted in the graph shown in Figure 10.2 indicate that the intervention increased on-task behavior well above baseline levels.

Line graphs can be created using software such as Microsoft Excel. For a more readily-accessible alternative, several different templates for creating graphs are provided in Appendix B. Unlike the VSSA Results Report Form, the **VSSI Graphing Templates** permit the instructor to plot and monitor performance following each work session or opportunity. Data collected via either the **VSSI Arranged Situations Template Data Sheet** or the **Additional Behaviors Sheets** can be graphed using one of these templates. Appendix B includes four different versions of the graphing template. The variation labeled, "Percentage," is used to graph data that is summarized as a percentage (e.g., percentage of opportunities, intervals, or responses). The variation labeled "Frequency" is used to graph data that is summarized as a frequency. The variation labeled "Rate" is used to graph data that is summarized as a rate. A slightly modified version of these templates, labeled "Blank," permits the instructor to individualize the vertical axis range. All of these summary options are described in more detail in this chapter.

An example graph using the **percentage-based version** of the **VSSI Graphing Template** is displayed in Figure 10.3. In the top section of the template, the instructor has written the target and relevant situation. The vertical axis displays percentage ranges (i.e., 0%–10%, 11%–20%) up to 100%, and the horizontal axis has spaces for the instructor to write the relevant session or observation numbers. For each session or observation, the instructor fills in the bubble that aligns with the percentage range that contains the obtained data.

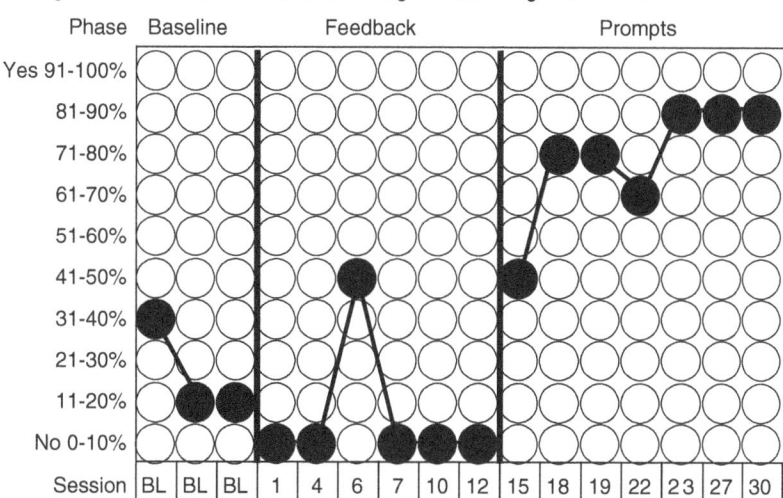

Figure 10.3 Example graph using the percentage-based version of the VSSI Graphing Template.

For the example in Figure 10.3, the learner emitted confirming statements in 33% of the opportunities that occurred during the first VSSA appointment (i.e., first baseline point; "BL"). As such, the instructor has filled in the bubble that aligns with the 31%–40% range for the first session plotted on the graph. Like the graph in Figure 10.2, the instructor has written "Baseline" over these data to indicate data collected prior to the VSSI (e.g., during the VSSA). The instructor also inserted horizontal lines to indicate the points at which they introduced new interventions, wrote the names of the interventions above the data, and used lines to connect each data point to the next one within each VSSI phase.

An example graph using the ***frequency-based version*** of the ***VSSI Graphing Template*** is displayed in Figure 10.4. Similar to the other version, the instructor has written the target and relevant situation at the top of the sheet. However, instead of percentage ranges, the vertical axis on the frequency-based version displays the numbers 0–20. Thus, this template permits the instructor to graph data up to a maximum of 20 responses per session or observation. If the learner is likely to emit more than 20 responses during any observation, the instructor should use the "Blank" version of the template to include a higher range of potential values on the vertical axis. Like the percentage-based version, the horizontal axis has spaces for the instructor to write the relevant session or observation numbers. In the example, the instructor has graphed frequency-based data on the number of

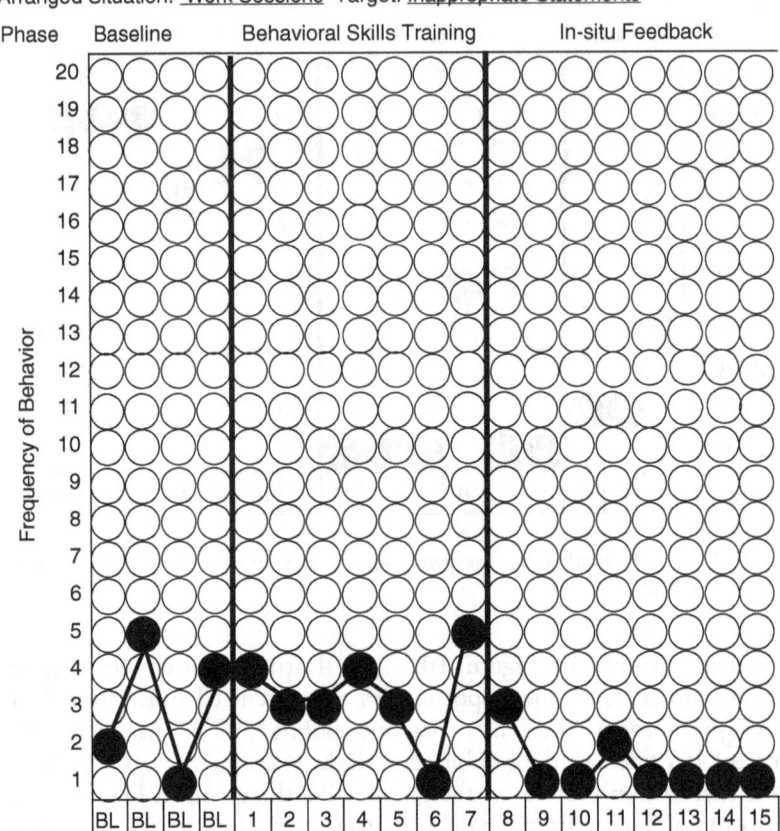

Figure 10.4 Example graph using the frequency-based version of the VSSI Graphing
Template.

inappropriate statements that occurred during work sessions, starting with
the VSSA (labeled "BL") and when the learner received two interventions
(BST, followed by in-situ feedback).

The potential advantages of converting data on frequency to rate were
discussed in Chapter 6. Recall that this requires the instructor to divide
the number of times that the behavior occurred by the total duration of
the observation or session. Calculating rate is desirable during the VSSI
when evaluating levels of responding across varied observation lengths.
The **rate-based version** of the **VSSI Graphing Template** is identical to
the frequency-based version displayed in Figure 10.4, with the exception
of the pre-filled values that appear next to the vertical axis. For this
template, the values range from 0 to 5 responses per minute. If those
values are not appropriate for a behavior, the instructor should use the

"Blank" version of the template to include a different range of potential values for the vertical axis numbers.

An example graph using the rate-based version of the **VSSI Graphing Template** is displayed in Figure 10.5. In this graph, data on inappropriate statements from Figure 10.4 were converted to a rate (responses per minute) by dividing the frequency in each session by the duration of each session. For illustrative purposes, suppose that the session times varied between 5 minutes and 15 minutes. Comparing the graphic displays in Figures 10.4 and 10.5 reveals similarities in the pattern of responding across the two displays. However, the instructor might draw slightly different conclusions about the effectiveness of the first intervention, BST, when inspecting the data in Figure 10.4 versus Figure 10.5. That is, compared to the baseline, the frequency of inappropriate statements seemed unchanged after the learner

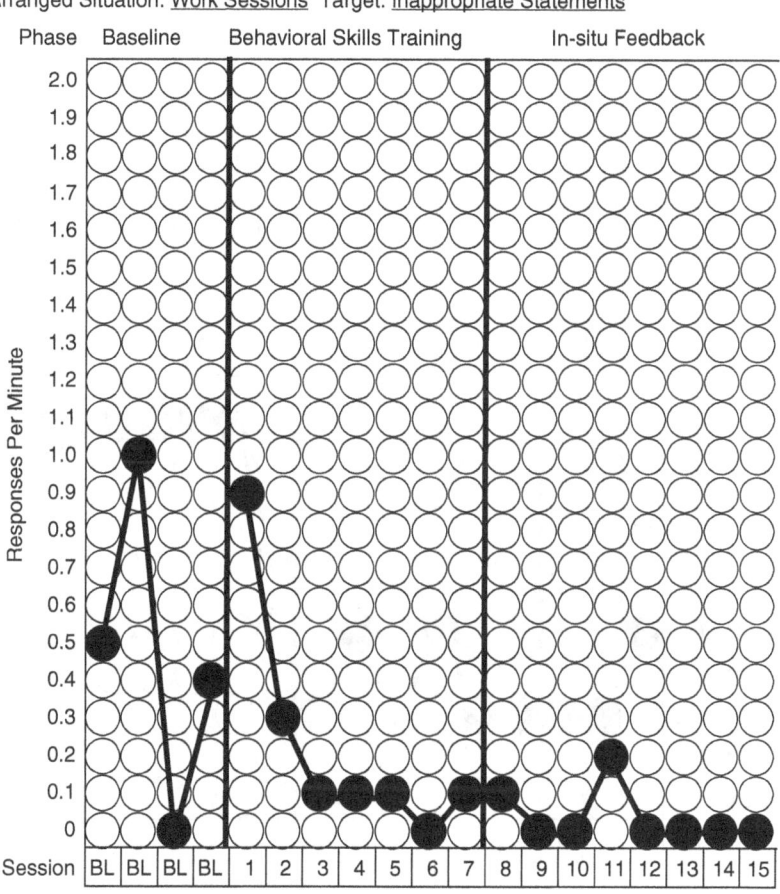

Figure 10.5 Example graph using the rate-based version of the VSSI Graphing Template.

received BST (Figure 10.4). However, after adjusting for the different session lengths, the data in Figure 10.5 suggest that BST was somewhat effective in reducing inappropriate statements.

Graphing Data from the Arranged Situations Data Sheet

As described previously, the instructor has the option to collapse across multiple targeted responses within the same opportunity or to examine each individual response separately when summarizing data collected using the **Arranged Situations Data Sheet**. For example, possible learner responses when they encounter broken or missing materials include (a) searching for materials in the supply cabinet, (b) finding the materials in the cabinet (if present), (c) seeking assistance from the supervisor (if needed), and (d) emitting an appropriate statement of help. The instructor could determine the percentage of possible responses (a)–(d) that the learner completed correctly each time they encountered missing or broken materials and then plot this percentage on a single graph. Figure 10.6 illustrates this approach using the percentage-based version of the **VSSI Graphing Template**:

Alternatively, the instructor could create individual graphs for each targeted response and report the outcome for each opportunity using a "yes"/"no" format in order to monitor the learner's progress in acquiring each response. As noted previously, this approach would readily reveal if

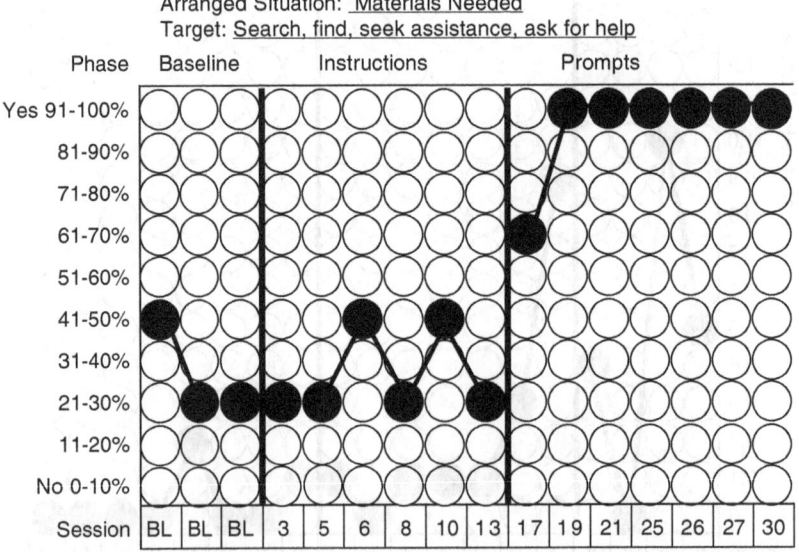

Figure 10.6 Example graph of data on correct responses in the materials-needed situation using the percentage-based version of the VSSI Graphing Template.

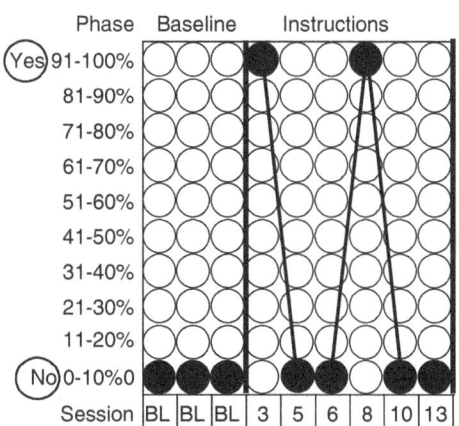

Arranged Situation: <u>Materials Needed</u> Target: <u>Ask for help</u>

Figure 10.7 Example graph of data collected on one targeted response in the materials-needed situation using the yes/no format of the VSSI Graphing Template.

the learner is having difficulty with certain responses. For example, the graph shown in Figure 10.6 indicates that the learner continued to perform some responses incorrectly after receiving spoken and written instructions, but it does not indicate if the learner struggled to acquire certain responses. The **percentage-based version** of the **VSSI Graphing Template** includes a yes/no format on the vertical axis (with "Y" aligning to 100% on the axis and "N" aligning to 0% on the axis). This permits the instructor to plot each response separately, as illustrated in Figure 10.7. This graph readily shows that the learner was struggling to learn how to emit an appropriate help statement. In this case, the instructor could focus on this particular response with additional interventions in the VSSI hierarchy.

Graphing Data from the Additional Behavior Data Sheets

When graphing data collected using one or more of the **Additional Behavior Data Sheets**, the instructor will have all four format options of the **VSSI Graphing Template** described previously. The most appropriate format will depend on the data sheet that the instructor uses (i.e., opportunity-based, interval-based, or frequency-based formats). The "Percentage" graphing format is used for opportunity- or interval-based recording, and the "Frequency" or "Rate" graphing formats are used for frequency-based recording. As noted previously, the instructor should graph the data on a session-by-session (or observation-by-observation) basis, or at a maximum, collapse across small groups of sessions or observations (e.g., daily sessions) for the purpose of monitoring performance over time.

Illustrative examples of graphing data from the additional behavior data sheets are provided in the next section and with the cases presented in Chapter 12.

Making Data-Based Decisions During the VSSI: Case Example

Before starting the VSSI, the instructor should determine how they plan to summarize and graph the data collected during the VSSI. They then begin the graphing process by plotting the baseline data for each targeted skill. With the initial VSSI plan in hand, the instructor is now ready to start the VSSI. As discussed in Chapters 8 and 9, the instructor makes decisions during the VSSI based on the learner's goals, the desired levels of performance (i.e., acquisition criteria), and the criteria for modifying the intervention if the learner does not make adequate progress (i.e., the intervention-change criteria). To do so effectively, the instructor should graph the learner's performance immediately after each work session or opportunity to respond or as frequently as possible.

Returning to John, the case example described in prior chapters, helps to illustrate this approach. In Chapter 9, John's instructor, Charise, started the VSSI with the work sessions shown in Table 10.1.

Charise decided to collapse the data collected for the two targeted responses (seeks assistance and asks for help) in each arranged situation and plot the outcome of each situation (vague instructions and time pressure) on separate graphs. Thus, for each session, Charise plotted 0% if John did not engage in either behavior correctly, 50% if he engaged in one of the two behaviors correctly, and 100% if he engaged in both of the behaviors correctly using the percentage-based format of the *VSSI Graphing Template*.

As described in Chapter 9, John did not seek assistance from or ask Charise for help when he received vague instructions in the first two sessions. She plotted this outcome, along with the associated baseline data from his VSSA, as shown in Figure 10.8. Thus, the next time that she introduced the vague-instructions situation (the 4th planned work session; see Table 10.2), she preceded it with BST because her change criterion was two sessions in a row with no improvement.

Table 10.1 First three sessions of John's VSSI plan

Session #	Target(s)	Intervention	Situation(s)
1	Seeks assistance; Asks for help	Written/Spoken Instructions	Vague Instructions
2	Seeks assistance; Asks for help	Written/Spoken Instructions	Vague Instructions
3	Seeks assistance; Asks for help	Written/Spoken Instructions	Time Pressure

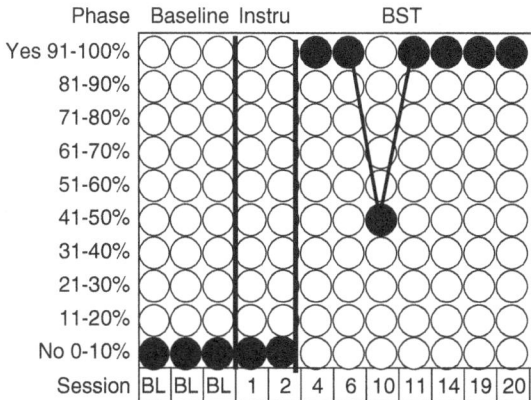

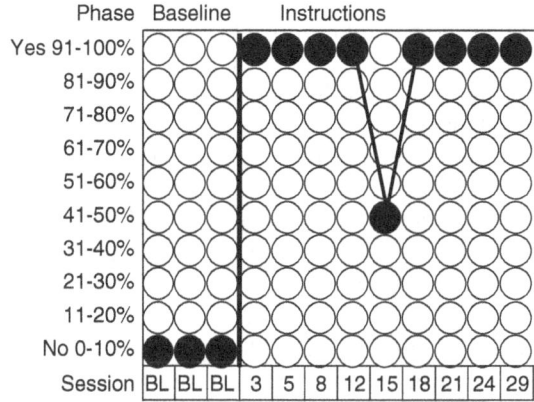

Figure 10.8 Graphs displaying John's data on seeking assistance and asking for help during the vague-instructions situation (top graph) and time-pressure situation (bottom graph).

In the third session, Charise arranged the time-pressure situation, and John immediately engaged in the correct responses (see bottom graph of Figure 10.8). John again responded correctly in the fourth session after receiving BST for the vague-instructions situation, as shown in the top graph of Figure 10.8. As shown in Table 10.2, Charise continued to evaluate his performance during these situations and also arranged the supervisor-unavailable situation so that she could evaluate the effects of written and spoken instructions on the associated target (i.e., working on other tasks).

Table 10.2 Next three sessions of John's VSSI plan

Session #	Target(s)	Intervention	Situation(s)
4	Seeks assistance; Asks for help	BST	Vague Instructions
5	Seeks assistance; Asks for help	N/A	Time Pressure
	Works on other tasks	Written/Spoken Instructions	Supervisor Unavailable
6	Seeks assistance; Asks for help;	N/A	Vague Instructions
	Works on other tasks	Written/Spoken Instructions	Supervisor Unavailable

John continued to perform at 100% with the exception of two work sessions (#10 and #15) during the vague-instructions and time-pressure situations as shown in the graphs in Figure 10.8.

As described in Chapter 9, Charise then introduced interventions for his two remaining targets, making confirming statements and acknowledging feedback, while occasionally evaluating his other targets. John had the opportunity to make confirming statements when he received new task instructions and when he received feedback. Charise decided to plot data for this behavior on different graphs because John could easily perform differently during these two distinct situations. For confirming understanding of new task instructions, Charise used the yes/no format of the graphing template to plot whether he engaged in the target for each opportunity.

The other target, acknowledging feedback, also should occur when his supervisor gives him feedback. Charise decided to combine the data collected for the two targeted responses that are associated with feedback (acknowledging feedback and confirming understanding) and plot them on a single graph. As such, John received 0% if he engaged in neither response, 50% if he engaged in one of the two responses correctly, and 100% if he engaged in both of the responses correctly. Charise created additional graphs for these targets using data from his VSSA for the baseline and also continued to graph the data for his other targets.

Figure 10.9 shows Charise's two graphs for these final targeted skills. The top graph shows whether or not he emitted a confirming statement each time he received a new task instruction (i.e., yes/no format). For the baseline data on confirming statements, Charise plotted just the last 5 opportunities from the VSSA. She determined it was not necessary to plot all of the data on confirming statements that she gathered during the VSSA because his performance was fairly consistent across the assessment. The bottom graph shows the percentage of the two targeted responses (acknowledges feedback, confirms understanding) that John emitted correctly when his supervisor provided feedback during the VSSA (baseline) and after receiving spoken and written instructions during the VSSI.

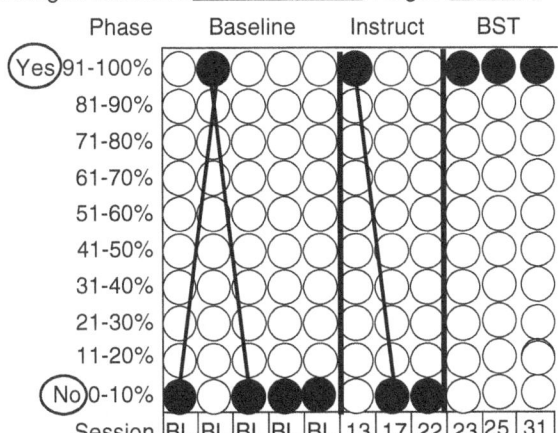

Arranged Situation: <u>New Instructions</u> Target: <u>Confirms</u>

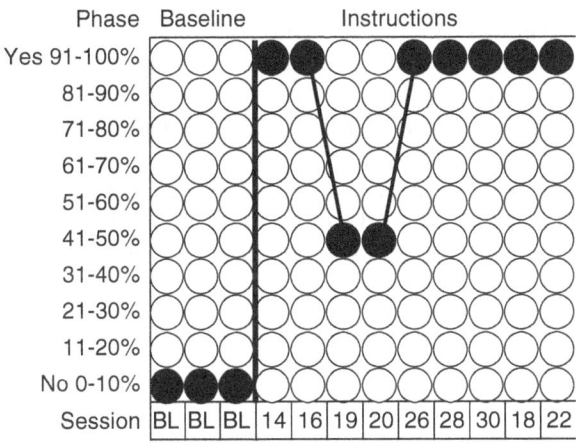

Arranged Situation: <u>Provided Feedback</u> Target: <u>Acknowledges,</u>
<u>Confirms,</u>

Figure 10.9 Graphs displaying John's data on confirming understanding of new task instructions (top graph) and acknowledging and confirming understanding of feedback (bottom graph).

Although John emitted a confirming statement to the first new instruction after receiving spoken and written instructions for this skill (session #13 in the top graph of Figure 10.9), he failed to do so in the next two opportunities (sessions #17 and #22). Thus, before she delivered a new task instruction again (session #23), Charise preceded it with BST because John had met the change criterion of two sessions in a row with no improvement. On the other hand, John's performance when he received

Table 10.3 John's acquisition goals

Behaviors	Acquisition Goal
Seeks assistance;	100% across 6 opportunities, 3 per arranged
Makes appropriate help statement	situation (vague instructions, time pressure)
Begins additional tasks when supervisor unavailable	Correct (i.e. "yes") across 3 opportunities
Makes confirming statement	Correct (i.e. "yes") across 6 opportunities, 3 per arranged situation (new task instruction, feedback)
Acknowledges feedback	Correct (i.e. "yes") across 3 opportunities

feedback (bottom graph in Figure 10.9) immediately improved and remained at 100% with spoken and written instructions. The exceptions were session #19, during which he did not acknowledge the feedback but did confirm his understanding of the instructions to fix his work, and #20, during which he acknowledged the feedback but did not confirm his understanding. Thus, Charise continued to monitor his performance rather than immediately introduce BST for this skill.

Charise continued to inspect all graphs to determine when John had met the acquisition criteria displayed in Table 10.3 (see also Chapter 8).

As shown in Figures 10.8 and 10.9, John met the acquisition goals for all of his targets. John needed only spoken and written instructions for all but a few of his targets. For those targets (seeks assistance and asks for help when given vague instructions and makes confirming statements when given new task instructions), John met his acquisition goal following BST.

In the next step, Charise continued to monitor John's performance to ensure that it generalized and maintained over time. This will be discussed in Chapter 11.

11 Maintenance and Generalization

In Chapter 10, our case example, John, met his acquisition goals fairly quickly when his instructor, Charise, introduced interventions based on her VSSI plan. However, John ultimately will not benefit from this intervention if the new skills fail to persist over time or if John does not perform them when he works in other settings or with supervisors other than Charise. Thus, as part of the VSSI, Charise should create a plan to help ensure that John's targeted responses will maintain over time and generalize beyond the context of the VSSI. As described in this chapter, Charise can draw from a number of research-based strategies to help John accomplish these goals.

Setting Goals for Maintenance and Generalization

Before identifying appropriate strategies, the instructor should collaborate with the learner to set appropriate maintenance and generalization goals. As with all behavioral goals, maintenance and generalization goals should include (a) the definition of a correct response (i.e., the criteria for considering a response as "correct" if different from that required during acquisition), (b) the desired level of performance, (c) the condition(s) under which the desired level of performance should occur (e.g., number/type of different settings, supervisors, or work tasks), and (d) the time period across which the learner is expected to maintain that level of performance. Compared to the initial acquisition goal, the instructor should consider a much lengthier time period when establishing the criteria for the maintenance goal (e.g., level of performance occurs across weeks or months rather than across work sessions or opportunities). In addition, as discussed in Chapter 8, it may be appropriate to set a less stringent, more practical goal for the desired level of performance during the maintenance period.

The following are some example maintenance and generalization goals for the same sample of targets provided in Chapter 8 when discussing possible acquisition goals:

DOI: 10.4324/9781003311935-11

- Target: Responding to Corrective Feedback

    Maintenance Goal: When Jerry is given corrective feedback, he will acknowledge the feedback by saying, "thank you," "I appreciate the feedback," or "I'm sorry about that" and then immediately correct his mistake on 75% of opportunities across two consecutive months.

    Generalization Goal: Jerry will acknowledge this corrective feedback across at least three different supervisors, two different work settings, and five different work tasks.

- Target: Responding Appropriately When Supervisor is Unavailable

    Maintenance Goal: When Shayla needs assistance to complete her work and discovers that her supervisor is unavailable, she will complete other work or ask a coworker for assistance on 80% of opportunities across three consecutive months.

    Generalization Goal: Shayla will respond correctly in at least three different work settings and during at least three different situations that require supervisor assistance.

- Target: On-Task Behavior

    Maintenance Goal: Drew will remain on-task for at least 70% of 20-minute intervals across five consecutive weeks.

    Generalization Goal: Drew will remain on-task for at least 70% of 20-minute intervals across at least six different work tasks, two different supervisors, and three different work settings.

- Target: Confirming Understanding

    Maintenance Goal: When assigned a new task, Octavia will confirm understanding of the task instructions by repeating the instructions and letting her supervisor know that she will complete the task on at least 50% of opportunities across four consecutive weeks.

    Generalization Goal: Octavia will confirm understanding of tasks across at least three different supervisors, two different work settings, and six different tasks.

Strategies to Promote Maintenance

The importance of long-term skill maintenance can not be overstated. Consistent performance, particularly independent of any support from supervisors, will increase employability and the likelihood of success on the job. One of the most important research-based strategies for promoting maintenance is to systematically fade out, or gradually remove, elements of that support. In particular, it is important to identify and reduce the learner's dependence on supports that might serve as a barrier to successful employment, such as a reliance on supervisor-delivered prompts, feedback, and reinforcement. Although it might be acceptable for an employee to need such support occasionally, employers value independence. Supervisors often do not have the capacity to provide a great deal of performance monitoring and oversight of employees' activities. The instructor should develop a plan for gradually fading these supports within the context of the VSSI to ensure the learner's success and promote independence.

In addition to fading out supports, the instructor should consider other strategies that may help promote long-term performance. As discussed in Chapters 3 and 9 (see "consequences for work completion"), some targeted behaviors may not maintain over the long run because they have subtle, delayed, or weak reinforcing consequences. Learners who have acquired these types of skills, even without in-situ support, likely would benefit from the periodic acknowledgment of their efforts. Thus, in some cases, it may be important to ensure that the learner continues to receive feedback, praise, or other reinforcers at least occasionally for correct responses. Finally, it may be beneficial to teach some learners how to manage their own behavior. All of these approaches are described in the following sections.

Fading Spoken and Written Instructions

In some cases, instructions may be highly effective but the learner continues to require occasional reviews of what they should do and why. The instructor can address this issue by providing these spoken instructions on a regular basis while gradually fading them over time. For example, the instructor or supervisor could begin by reducing the amount of reviews over time until the instructions take the form of a brief reminder (e.g., "Remember to find other work to do if I am too busy to help you with a problem."). If a reminder is effective, the instructor could reduce it even further (e.g., "Remember what to do when I am busy.") or pose a question for the learner to answer (e.g., "What should you do when I am too busy to help you with a problem?"). The instructor should ensure that the learner has frequent opportunities to perform the newly acquired skill while evaluating the effectiveness of these faded instructions. The instructor also may need to fade written instructions if the learner frequently references them in a manner that hinders the learner's success on the job. In this case, the instructor could remove parts of the written instructions gradually over time, as illustrated in Figure 11.1.

In the final fading step, the instructor would remove the paper from the work area.

Fading In-Situ Feedback

As recommended in Chapter 9, the instructor should provide in-situ feedback by informing the learner when they have performed a skill correctly (called "positive feedback") and when they have performed a skill incorrectly (called "corrective feedback"). When in-situ feedback is highly effective for a learner, the *corrective* aspect of the feedback will fade naturally over time.

Original

> If the supervisor interrupts your work to give you a new task:
>
> 1. Finish the new task.
> 2. Tell the supervisor you are done with the new task.
> 3. Finish the first task you were working on.

Fading Step 1

> If supervisor interrupts:
>
> 1. Finish new task.
> 2. Tell supervisor done.
> 3. Finish first task.

Fading Step 2:

> Interruption:
>
> 1. Finish new.
> 2. Tell supervisor.
> 3. Finish first

Fading Step 3

> Interrupt:
>
> 1. Finish.
> 2. Tell.
> 3. Finish.

Fading Step 4

> Interrupt:
>
> 1.
> 2.
> 3.

Figure 11.1 Example steps for fading written instructions.

That is, as the learner's correct responses increase over time, they will require less corrective feedback from the supervisor. The instructor will then need to fade the frequency of their *positive* feedback. It should be emphasized that the instructor should only decrease – not eliminate – their feedback for correct responses. Most everyone appreciates receiving praise periodically for good performance. Reducing the frequency of this praise will help ensure that the learner's performance maintains in the long run with just occasional supervisor input. One way to accomplish this goal is to provide positive feedback based on a gradually increasing number of correct responses. For example, the instructor could deliver positive feedback after every two correct responses, then after every three correct responses, and so on, until they reach a terminal feedback schedule. Alternatively, the instructor could base the delivery of feedback on a gradually increasing amount of time. For example, they could begin by providing positive feedback for at least one correct response every 30 minutes, then every 60 minutes, and so on. Regardless of whether the instructor fades the schedule based on the number of responses or the amount of time, they should continue to monitor performance very closely to ensure that it maintains during the fade.

The instructor should select the terminal schedule of feedback delivery by considering the expectations and practices of supervisors on current and potential job sites, as well as the frequency of feedback needed for the learner to achieve their maintenance goals. If the learner's performance falters unless feedback is delivered more frequently than that typically provided by supervisors on their current or eventual job placement, the instructor should attempt to work with these supervisors so that the learner can be successful. In particular, the instructor might explain what the learner needs and brainstorm with the supervisor ways for the learner to obtain this level of support.

Fading In-Situ Prompts

Embedded spoken, visual, and technology prompts can be highly effective in promoting the acquisition of new skills. However, it is important to ensure that the learner does not become dependent on any prompts that will hinder their employability or success on the job. Prompts that require the full attention of supervisors, particularly those that must be delivered "in the moment," are most likely to serve as barriers to independence. For this reason, it is important for the instructor to prioritize the types of prompts that they can fade easily from the work environment. The strategy for fading prompts depends on the modality and timing of the prompt. As discussed in Chapter 9, it can be beneficial if the instructor delivers the prompt before or immediately after the learner encounters the relevant situation. Although this may reduce the likelihood of an incorrect response, the instructor will need to gradually remove the prompt while ensuring that the learner's performance maintains.

The instructor can use several different strategies to fade spoken, visual, and technology prompts. First, the instructor could modify the timing of the prompt by gradually delaying its delivery. For example, instead of delivering a spoken or textual prompt immediately after the learner has completed a task (e.g., "Tell your supervisor, 'I'm done. What should I do next?'"), the instructor could wait for 20 seconds. This gives the learner an opportunity to respond correctly in the absence of the prompt.

The instructor could then delay the prompt even further by waiting for 40 seconds, then 60 seconds, and so on, until the learner begins to respond independently. This approach to prompt fading is called "progressive prompt delay." A similar strategy could be applied to technology-delivered prompts that occur at regular intervals (e.g., automated cell phone reminders to remain on-task). For example, the instructor could gradually increase the amount of time that elapses between each automated reminder (e.g., from every 10 minutes, to every 20 minutes, etc).

A different strategy is recommended if the learner tends to respond incorrectly before receiving a prompt. Instead of delaying the prompt, the instructor could gradually reduce the prompt itself over time or transition across different types of prompts. For example, spoken and textual prompts could be faded by simply reducing the amount of information provided, in a manner similar to that shown for spoken and written instructions earlier in this chapter. Pictures could be reduced in size or gradually lightened until they no longer provide discernible information. Figure 11.2 illustrates how an instructor could gradually reduce the amount of a spoken or textual prompt about notifying the supervisor of task completion

The instructor also might fade prompts by transitioning to a prompt that provides less assistance before attempting to completely eliminate prompts. For example, an instructor might start by modeling how to search the supply cabinet for additional materials (either in person or through videos) and then switch to gesturing towards the supply cabinet or providing a spoken prompt (e.g., "Where do you find more materials?"). Regardless of how the instructor fades the prompts, they should monitor the learner's performance to ensure that it continues to maintain during the fade. If responding falters, they should return to the previous fading steps and attempt to fade the prompts again.

Full prompt: "Tell your supervisor, 'I'm done. What should I do next?'"

    Fade 1: "Tell your supervisor: 'I'm done. What ____?'"

    Fade 2: "Tell your supervisor: 'I'm done. Wha ____?'"

    Fade 3: "Tell your supervisor: 'I'm done. _____'"

    Fade 4: "Tell your supervisor: 'I'm _____.'"

    Fade 5: "Tell your supervisor: '____'"

    Fade 6: "Tell your _____

    Fade 7: "Tell _____

Figure 11.2 Example steps for fading vocal or textual prompts.

Fading In-Situ Reinforcement

As noted in Chapter 9, some learners may be more successful in acquiring skills when the instructor provides tangible reinforcement along with positive feedback (e.g., "Nice asking for more materials!") for correct responses. These reinforcers, tailored to the preferences of the individual learner, include food, activities, work breaks, preferred work tasks, and tokens. Initially, it is recommended to deliver these reinforcers quite frequently until the learner meets their acquisition goals. Like feedback and prompts, however, the instructor will need to gradually reduce the frequency of reinforcement to help the learner achieve their long-term maintenance goals. The same approaches to fading feedback can be applied to reinforcement. That is, the instructor can deliver reinforcement after a gradually increasing number of correct responses or a gradually increasing period of time.

For example, after initially delivering reinforcement every time a learner notifies her of task completion, the instructor might begin to deliver reinforcement after every other notification, then after the third notification, and so on. At the same time, the instructor should continue to provide positive feedback (e.g., "Thank you for letting me know that you are done with the task.") following responses that do not produce tangible reinforcement. If the learner's response maintains when the instructor delivers reinforcement very infrequently, the instructor should then begin to fade the feedback as described previously. The ultimate goal of reinforcement fading is for the learner to maintain performance with just periodic recognition of their efforts. As noted previously, the learner is more likely to be successful if their skills maintain under a schedule of feedback or reinforcement delivery that is consistent with the practices of supervisors on current and potential job sites. However, the instructor may need to identify the least amount of feedback or reinforcement that is needed for the learner to achieve their maintenance goals. If this schedule exceeds typical practices on the job site despite attempts to gradually fade out this support, the instructor may need to identify a job site that would better match the learner's needs or advocate on behalf of the learner to ensure that they can secure this critical support.

The token system described in Chapter 9 provides additional considerations for fading. The instructor can fade the frequency of the token delivery by requiring more responses to earn a token, the frequency of the token exchange by increasing the length of time between opportunities to exchange the tokens for backup reinforcers, *or* the cost of the backup reinforcers. It is recommended to start by reducing the frequency of the token delivery. For example, suppose a learner receives one token every time they remain on task for 20 minutes and can exchange their tokens for backup reinforcers during every scheduled break. To begin the fading process, the instructor might deliver a token every time they remain on task for 30 minutes, then 40 minutes, and so on. As the instructor reduces the frequency of the token delivery, it will take longer for the learner to acquire enough tokens to purchase items from their reinforcer menu. Unless the instructor reduces the prices of the backup reinforcers, the learner will necessarily wait longer to receive the backup reinforcers because they will need more time to accumulate the amount needed for the exchange. For example, they may need to wait until the last break of the work day or the very end of the work day. Eventually, they may need to collect tokens across multiple days before accumulating enough for the exchange. This is likely the simplest approach for fading the token reinforcement system.

Arranging Periodic Reinforcement

The eloquent principle that behavior is a function of its consequences, as discussed in Chapter 3, provides the foundation for most of the recommendations in this book. Behaviors that do not serve a purpose for the learner are unlikely to maintain over the long run. For this reason, instructors are encouraged to ensure that learners continue to receive at least periodic recognition of their efforts even after fading in-situ feedback and reinforcement. Even learners who initially acquire skills during the VSSI with relatively simple interventions, such as spoken and written instructions, may benefit from this approach.

For all learners, it is important to consider the reinforcing consequences that might maintain performance in the job setting beyond any support arranged by the instructor. As noted in Chapters 3 and 9, many social skills (e.g., asking for help) will result in immediate natural consequences (e.g., getting the help needed) that should ensure that performance persists on the job. However, other targeted behaviors, such as acknowledging feedback, making confirming statements, and orienting to listeners when speaking, have subtle, delayed, or weak natural consequences. Certainly, these behaviors can improve social relationships with supervisors and coworkers. However, these consequences may develop very gradually and may not be readily apparent or highly effective as a reinforcer for the learner.

To better determine whether the learner's behavior is likely to receive effective, naturalistic reinforcement on the job, the instructor should address the following questions for every targeted skill:

- What typically happens when workers engage in this behavior or when they fail to engage in this behavior? How do people (i.e., supervisors and coworkers) typically respond to the behavior?
- What are the immediate and delayed consequences of the behavior?
- Does the learner enjoy these types of consequences? Would the consequences function as reinforcers for their behavior even if they are fairly delayed?

A form to help guide the instructor through these questions, called the "Identifying Natural Consequences Worksheet," is provided in

Appendix A. The case example at the end of this chapter also illustrates this process.

If it isn't clear that a behavior will result in reinforcing consequences for the learner or that the consequences will be too delayed, the instructor should try to ensure that the learner receives at least some type of recognition for their efforts. This recognition should be in a form that is reinforcing to the learner and, if needed, occur fairly immediately after the behavior is performed. Chapter 3 discussed ways to identify reinforcers for learners.

Teaching Self-Management

A final recommended strategy that may be appropriate for some learners is to teach them how to manage their own behavior. This also may be helpful when the instructor cannot ensure that the learner will continue to receive recognition for their efforts. The goal is to replace the supervisor's support with the learner's own self-management strategies. When combined with the fading techniques described previously in this chapter, this approach may help ensure the learner's performance persists over time while they achieve more independence on the job. Such an outcome will increase their value to potential employers and their likely success in the workplace. Self-management typically includes goal-setting, self-monitoring, self-evaluation, and self-reinforcement, as described in the following sections:

*   Goal-Setting and Self-Monitoring: With the instructor's assistance, the learner establishes daily or weekly performance goals and a plan for tracking their own performance while on the job so they can determine their success. The goals typically differ from the learner's maintenance goals, which target desired levels of performance across extended periods of time. Because the learner will be monitoring and evaluating their own performance, the goals should tie directly to this monitoring system. Self-monitoring requires some type of data collection system that would be practical for the learner to transport and use while completing their work responsibilities. The data collection system might involve the use of paper and pencil (e.g., checklists), tally counters, or electronic devices (e.g., cell phones or tablets) with specially-designed apps (e.g., Countee).

For example, suppose a learner's target is to respond appropriately when their supervisor gives them corrective feedback. They might set a daily goal to respond correctly each time they receive feedback. They could then easily track whether they respond correctly or incorrectly by using a data sheet on a clipboard located in their work area, as illustrated below. Whenever their supervisor gives them feedback, they would indicate whether they responded correctly by placing a mark in the "yes" or "no" column, as shown in Figure 11.3.

When my supervisor gave me feedback, I thanked them and corrected my work.		
Day	YES	NO
Monday	//	/
Tuesday		///

Figure 11.3 Example self-monitoring sheet.

As another example, suppose a learner's target is to confirm their understanding (e.g., say "Got it!") when their supervisor gives them an instruction. They might set a goal to confirm their understanding of instructions at least three times each day. They could affix a hand tally counter to their belt loop or to a lanyard worn around the neck and press the counter each time they make a confirming statement. The counter would then give them a running total of their confirming statements each day.

As a final example, suppose a learner's target is to stay on task during a 3-hour daily work shift. One possible self-monitoring strategy is to arrange for their cell phone to buzz or vibrate every 20 minutes. Using a data sheet like the one shown in Figure 11.4, they would circle "yes" or "no" if they are on task when the cell phone emits the signal. They might set a daily goal of remaining on task for at least 8 of the 20-minute intervals.

- Self-Evaluation and Self-Reinforcement. Goal-setting and self-monitoring provide the opportunity for the learner to recognize and reward their own success. Thus, with the instructor's assistance, the learner should develop a plan for evaluating their own performance data and determining whether they have met their goal. For example, the goal could be prominently displayed on their data sheet or a card placed in their wallet. At the end of each work shift, the learner should examine their performance data and compare it to their goal. If the goal is met, they could then arrange their own reward or share their findings with family, coworkers, or friends who will celebrate their success and perhaps provide rewards, as well. A self-evaluation sheet, as illustrated in Figure 11.5, may be helpful for some learners.

When cell phone buzzes, circle "yes" if working and "no" if not working									
YES	YES	YES	YES	YES	YES	YES	YES	YES	YES
NO	NO	NO	NO	NO	NO	NO	NO	NO	NO

Figure 11.4 Example self-monitoring sheet.

Daily Goal: Remain on Task for At Least 8 20-minute Intervals
Number of times "YES" circled: _____
Is this number larger than 7? If yes, reward yourself with a soda or chips!

Figure 11.5 Example self-evaluation sheet.

The instructor should assist the learner to brainstorm various ways they can reward themselves when they meet their goals. For example, they might treat themselves to a special snack or activity after work.

Teaching learners to self-manage requires careful instructional planning. Some learners may need quite a bit of training and practice to master these self-management strategies. Behavioral skills training, consisting of instructions, modeling, and practice with feedback as described in Chapter 9, can be highly effective for preparing learners to set goals, self-monitor, evaluate their own performance, and reward their success. Additional resources for teaching self-management skills can be found in the reference list at the end of this chapter (Lancioni & O'Reilly, 2001; Najdowski, 2017; Palmen & Didden, 2012; Wheeler et al., 1988).

Strategies to Promote Generalization

While it is important for skills to persist over time, the learner will not be successful if the skills acquired with the support of the instructor during the VSSI do not transfer when the learner is working in other settings, with other supervisors, and on other tasks. This outcome is particularly important when the instructor implements the VSSI in a simulated, or "training," work environment in order to prepare the learner for employment. Research has identified a number of strategies that the instructor can embed within the VSSI to increase the likelihood of generalization (Stokes et al., 1977; Stokes & Osnes, 1989). Some of these recommended strategies are described in the following sections.

Use Multiple Exemplars

The most common strategy for promoting generalization is to ensure that the learner practices the skills while experiencing a variety of stimuli that might be encountered on the job. These "stimuli" include the various tasks and materials needed to complete the tasks; features of the setting or location (e.g., large versus small room, at a table versus desk, with others versus alone); and characteristics of the supervisor (e.g., man versus woman, short versus tall; stern versus friendly). Including as many exemplars of these stimuli as possible in the VSSI may be highly beneficial for the learner.

Instructors, however, will necessarily have constraints on the number of different exemplars and/or varying situations that they can arrange during the VSSI. Furthermore, research has not clearly identified the minimum number of exemplars needed to promote generalization. The ideal number of exemplars likely depends on the learner. Thus, it is simply recommended to include as much variation within the VSSI as possible. This might be accomplished by (a) occasionally recruiting other people to serve as the supervisor, (b) assigning a variety of tasks and responsibilities to the learner, (c) arranging for the learner to work in different rooms and/or with different peers, and (d) modifying other physical features of the work environment (e.g., changing the position of furniture and needed supplies).

Incorporate Common Stimuli

Another frequently recommended strategy is to modify the training environment so that it resembles the planned work environment as much as possible. This approach is useful when the instructor is conducting the VSSI separately from the learner's current or potential job site and can identify and access work-related exemplars from those sites. Information about the actual job site forms the basis of the exemplars incorporated into the VSSI. Research on generalization indicates that the learner will be more likely to transfer new skills from the VSSI to the job site if the two environments contain enough similarities. Suppose, for example, that a learner desires a job in a grocery store, where they would like to stock shelves and bag merchandise. The instructor might visit local grocery stores to gather information about common features of floor supervisors, products, shelving units, price tags, bags, etc. The instructor could then incorporate similar materials (products, shelving, price tags, bags, supervisors' style of clothing, and nametags) into the simulated work environment. This strategy also illustrates the benefit of conducting the VSSA and VSSI on existing job sites if the learner is currently employed.

Incorporate Mediators of Generalization

Another generalization strategy that may be more practical is to establish some type of stimulus as a prompt or reminder for engaging in the correct response and then arrange for the learner to transport this stimulus to the workplace. These stimuli can take the form of visual or technology-delivered prompts described in Chapter 9, including text, pictures, or automated reminders that are delivered via cell phones or tablets. For example, during the VSSI for one of our learners, we provided text prompts on a letter-size sheet of paper that displayed different ways that hecould ask for help from his supervisor when he didn't understand how to do a task (e.g., "Can you show me how?" "Can you demonstrate it?" "I need an example.") Because he found these text prompts so helpful in the training setting, we realized that they might be useful for promoting generalization of the skill to his actual job site. Instead of fading the text prompts, we ensured that the learner continued to use them while giving him a variety of new tasks in different rooms of the training center. However, we also considered the practicality and accessibility of these text prompts in light of his desire to work as a member of the janitorial staff at a sports arena. This job would require him to move around the arena, so we were concerned that the letter-size sheet of paper would not be practical or easily accessible to him on the job site. Thus, we printed the text prompts on a small, laminated card that could be affixed to a key chain that he already wore at his waist. The learner then practiced using this card when he needed to ask for help with a task.

The self-management strategies described previously in this chapter also produce similar "mediators" of generalization that the learner can transport across settings. This includes the self-monitoring sheets, devices (e.g., tally counter), and self-evaluation forms. The presence of these stimuli may "cue" the learner to perform the skills despite new locations, tasks, people, or other situations encountered on the job. Thus, these self-management strategies may help promote both maintenance and generalization.

Case Example

Let's now return to the case example, John, to illustrate the application of the maintenance and generalization strategies described in this chapter. In collaboration with John, Charise added goals for maintenance and generalization (shown in the right two columns of Table 11.1) to his existing acquisition goals.

Although John's goal for all of his targets during acquisition was to perform correctly on 100% of opportunities, Charise recognized the need to select more practical criteria for long-term performance. It is not critical for

Table 11.1 John's acquisition, maintenance, and generalization goals

Behaviors	Acquisition	Maintenance	Generalization
Make confirming statement	100% across 6 opportunities, 3 per arranged situation	75% of opportunities across 2 weeks	3 different people, two locations
Acknowledge feedback	100% across 3 opportunities	75% of opportunities acrioss 2 weeks	3 different people, two locations
Seek assistance	100% across 6 opportunities, 3 per arranged situation	90% of opportunities across 2 weeks	3 different people, two locations
Make appropriate help statement	100% across 6 opportunities, 3 per arranged situation	90% of opportunities across 2 weeks	3 different people, two locations
Begin additional tasks when supervisor unavailable	100% across 3 opportunities	90% of opportunities across 2 weeks	3 different people, two locations

employees to emit confirming statements or to acknowledge feedback every single time there is an opportunity to do so; thus, Charise suggested a maintenance goal level of 75%. On the other hand, John may be unsuccessful if he does not seek assistance or ask for help when he encounters a problem that prevents work completion and if he does not remain on task even when the supervisor is unavailable. Thus, she and John select a somewhat higher maintenance goal for these behaviors, targeting a performance level of 90%. For his generalization goals, both John and Charise believe that it would be most practical and important for him to engage in these behaviors with at least three different people and in at least two different locations.

After establishing the goals, Charise considered potential strategies to increase the likelihood that John's performance would maintain over time and generalize across people and locations. As described in Chapter 10, John met the acquisition goals for his targeted behaviors when he received the interventions shown in Table 11.2.

Charise began by considering the targets that John successfully acquired after receiving spoken and written instructions (acknowledging feedback, seeking assistance and asking for help when given time pressure, and beginning additional tasks when the supervisor is unavailable). In considering her plan to ensure the maintenance of these behaviors, Charise answered the following questions:

Spoken/Written Instructions:
• Does John continue to rely on the written instructions?

   • Response: Yes, when his supervisor is unavailable, John frequently consults his instructions before working on additional tasks. He does not consult his instructions for the other targeted behaviors.

• Does he need periodic reminders to perform the skills?

   • Response: No, thus far, John continues to perform the targeted skills without reminders during the VSSI.

Because John continued to depend on the written instructions when his supervisor was not available, Charise considered whether it would be

Table 11.2 Intervention needed for John to meet his acquisition goal for each targeted skill

Behavior	Intervention(s)
Make confirming statement	BST
Acknowledge feedback	Spoken/Written Instructions
Seek assistance;	BST (Vague Instructions);
ask for help	Spoken/Written Instructions (Time Pressure)
Begin additional tasks	Spoken/Written Instructions

beneficial to fade out the instruction sheet. On the one hand, Charise wanted to increase John's independence and, hence, his employability. On the other hand, John had been keeping the instructions on a small piece of paper that he placed near his work area, and his reliance on these instructions seemed inconspicuous. His use of the written instructions did not interfere with his performance. Furthermore, Charise thought that these instructions might help John respond appropriately when this situation arose on future job sites. In fact, Charise recognized that the instruction sheet could serve as a "mediator of generalization," helping to promote the transfer of this skill across settings. Thus, instead of fading out the instruction sheet, Charise decided to incorporate it into her plans to promote generalization.

Next, Charise considered whether John would be likely to receive effective, naturalistic reinforcement for engaging in these behaviors on the job. To help make this determination, Charise answered the following questions for each target behavior with the responses shown in Tables 11.3 and 11.4:

• What typically happens when workers engage in this behavior or fail to engage in this behavior? How do people (i.e., supervisors and coworkers) typically respond to the behavior? What are the immediate and delayed consequences of the behavior?

Table 11.3 Charise's responses to questions about naturalistic consequences for John's targeted skills

Behavior	Answers
Make confirming statement	Immediate: The supervisor will move on and permit John to start the new task; no other immediate consequence is apparent. If John fails to confirm the instruction, the supervisor might ask John if he understands. Delayed: John's relationship with his supervisor might benefit over time if he consistently confirms understanding of instructions.
Acknowledge feedback	Immediate: No immediate consequences, regardless of whether John acknowledges the feedback. Delayed: John's relationship with his supervisor might benefit over time if he consistently acknowledges feedback.
Seek assistance; ask for help	Immediate: The supervisor or coworker will provide the requested help or assistance. John will not get the help if he doesn't request it. Delayed: John may lose his job if he doesn't do his work correctly because he consistently fails to request help.
Begin additional tasks	Immediate: No immediate consequences if he begins additional tasks. If John does not begin additional tasks, his supervisor might correct him for taking an unauthorized break. Delayed: John may be more likely to retain his job if he remains on task.

- Does John enjoy these types of consequences? Would the consequences function as reinforcers for their behavior even if they are fairly delayed?

Table 11.4 Charise's responses to questions about whether the naturalistic consequences for John's targeted skills would serve as reinforcers

Consequences	Answers
The supervisor moves on and permits John to start the new task	John enjoys working so the immediate consequence seems reinforcing.
Improved relationships	This consequence may be too subtle or delayed to be effective for John.
Obtains help needed	John finds it reinforcing to finish his work; thus, he likely would value the help.
Increased likelihood of job retention	John is really eager to do well on the job and to maintain employment. He will avoid negative evaluations by staying on task. Thus, this consequence is a natural reinforcer for John to begin additional tasks when his supervisor is unavailable.

Charise's answers to these questions suggested that the typical consequences for two of John's targeted behaviors (confirming understanding and acknowledging feedback) may not maintain his performance. She believed that John would benefit from additional planning to ensure that he continues to make confirming statements and acknowledge feedback. Although she could arrange for future supervisors to periodically praise John for engaging in these behaviors, Charise believed that John would benefit more if she taught him how to manage his own behavior. As discussed previously in the chapter, Charise needed to teach John how to set goals, monitor his behavior, evaluate his performance, and deliver reinforcement when he met his goals. She met with John to share her suggestion and, together, they prepared a plan for his self-management training. Because John's future employers had not yet been identified, Charise helped John develop the following plan for managing his own behavior during practice sessions at the therapeutic clinic.

Goal-Setting and Self-Monitoring

The first step was to identify goals for confirming understanding of new task instructions and acknowledging feedback. To keep things simple for John, Charise suggested that he set a goal to make at least one of these statements (confirming or acknowledging) at least one time during each work shift. Next, they considered possible ways for John to track this performance while working. John wanted something that would be inconspicuous and easy to carry around. John typically kept loose change in his right front pocket, and this gave Charise an idea. She suggested that John move one of the coins to his left pocket each time he confirmed understanding of an instruction or acknowledged feedback. When he returns home after work, he could record a YES or NO on a self-monitoring data sheet to indicate whether there was at least one coin in his left pocket that day.

Self-Evaluation and Self-Reinforcement

The final step was for John to develop a plan for determining whether he had met his goal and, if so, to reward his own success. Charise suggested that initially John reward himself as soon as he gets home if he recorded a YES on the self-monitoring sheet. John and Charise then brainstormed possible reinforcers for John by having him complete the reinforcer survey provided in Appendix A. John decided that he would watch a favorite YouTube video if he recorded a YES on the sheet. If the self-monitoring plan seems effective, Charise will eventually suggest that John establish weekly goals.

After establishing a plan for promoting maintenance, Charise considered strategies to ensure that John's performance in the clinic transferred to actual job sites. Charise decided to incorporate multiple exemplar training into his practice sessions at the clinic by recruiting several of her coworkers to occasionally arrange the relevant situations (e.g., provide feedback, deliver a time pressure statement) and for John to sometimes work in different locations at the clinic (e.g., in the kitchen, front office, conference room). She also had John practice transporting his written instructions to different locations so that he could rely on this "mediator of generalization."

Reference List

Lancioni & O'Reilly (2001). Self-management of instruction cues for occupation: Review of studies with people with severe and profound developmental disabilities. *Research in Developmental Disabilities, 22*(1), 41–65. 10.1016/S0891-4222(00)00063-9

Najdowski, A. C. (2017). *Flexible and focused: Teaching executive function skills to individuals with autism and attention disorders.* Academic Press.

Palmen, A., & Didden, R. (2012). Task engagement in young adults with high-functioning autism spectrum disorders: Generalization effects of behavioral skills training. *Research in Autism Spectrum Disorders, 6*(4), 1377–1388. 10.1016/j.rasd.2010.01.012

Stokes, T. F., & Baer, D. M. (1977). An implicit technology of generalization. *Journal of Applied Behavior Analysis, 10*(2), 349–36.

Stokes, T. F., & Osnes, P. G. (1989). An operant pursuit of generalization. *Behavior Therapy, 20*(3), 337–355.

Wheeler, J. J., Bates, P., Marshall, K. J., & Miller, S. R. (1988). Teaching appropriate social behaviors to a young man with moderate mental retardation in a supported competitive employment setting. *Education and Training in Mental Retardation, 23*(2), 105–116. https://www.jstor.org/stable/23878434

12 VSSI Case Examples

Chapter 7 introduced four case examples and described their VSSAs. In this chapter, we return to each case example to illustrate their VSSIs.

Case Example #1: Sergio

Sergio is a 16-year-old student with autism and moderate intellectual disabilities who receives special education services in a public high school. Sergio communicates using the symbol-based software application Proloquo2Go installed on an iPad, which he carries with him in a bag strapped around his shoulders.

Sergio is receiving work experience in the cafeteria and school store on his high school campus. Sergio's teacher and his parents would like to prepare Sergio for his first part-time job in the community by expanding his goals to include relevant social-communication and problem-solving targets. His teacher, Trina, conducted the VSSA within the context of his vocational training on campus. After considering the results of the VSSA and factors related to Sergio's likely initial job placement, they decided to prioritize teaching Sergio to seek assistance and communicate using his iPad when he needs materials and when he has completed his tasks. They also would like Sergio to learn how to transition across multiple tasks without assistance. Now, Trina must complete the steps needed to prepare for the VSSI.

Step 1: Set Goals

Trina's first step is to establish goals for the acquisition, maintenance, and generalization of the targeted skills. In collaboration with Sergio and his parents, she sets the following goals:

Acquisition Goals
- Target: Responding Appropriately When Materials Are Needed
  Goal: When Sergio discovers that he does not have all of the materials needed to complete his task, he will approach his supervisor

DOI: 10.4324/9781003311935-12

within two minutes and press the "help" icon on his iPad across six consecutive opportunities.

- Target: Responding Appropriately When Task is Completed
  Goal: When Sergio has completed all of his assigned tasks and does not know what to do next, he will approach his supervisor within two minutes and press the "finished" icon on his iPad across six consecutive opportunities.

- Target: Transitioning Across Multiple Tasks
  Goal: When given up to three tasks to complete in a particular sequence, Sergio will begin each new task within one minute of completing the previous one until he has completed all of the assigned tasks across six consecutive opportunities.

Maintenance and Generalization Goals

- Target: Responding Appropriately When Materials Are Needed
  Maintenance Goal: When Sergio discovers that he does not have all of the materials needed to complete his task, he will approach his supervisor within two minutes and press the "help" icon on his iPad on at least 90% of opportunities across six weeks.

  Generalization Goal: Sergio will respond correctly across at least five different tasks, two different supervisors, and four different work locations.

- Target: Responding Appropriately When Task is Completed
  Maintenance Goal: When Sergio has completed all of his assigned tasks and does not know what to do next, he will approach his supervisor within two minutes and press the "finished" icon on his iPad on at least 90% of opportunities across six weeks.

  Generalization Goal: Sergio will respond correctly across at least five different tasks, two different supervisors, and four different work locations.

- Target: Transitioning Across Multiple Tasks
  Maintenance Goal: When given up to three tasks to complete in a particular sequence, Sergio will begin each new task within one minute of completing the previous one until he has completed all of the assigned tasks on 80% of opportunities across six weeks.

  Generalization Goal: Sergio will respond correctly across at least four different task sequences, two different supervisors, and four different work locations.

As discussed in Chapters 8 and 9, Trina also must establish a criterion for modifying the intervention (i.e., progressing to more intensive training) during the VSSI if Sergio does not make adequate progress. Based on Sergio's prior learning history, Trina decides that she will modify the intervention for a target if Sergio does not show any improvement in that target after four consecutive opportunities. She also plans to modify the intervention if Sergio does not meet the acquisition criterion for a target after 24 total opportunities. She included this latter criterion because Sergio's performance is sometimes quite variable. Thus, he might show some improvement but still fail to acquire the skill in a timely manner. By including a criterion based on the total number of opportunities without meeting the criterion, Trina hopes to increase the efficiency of the VSSI. The following summarizes her criteria:

Intervention-Change Criteria
- No improvement across four consecutive opportunities
- Failure to meet the acquisition goal after 24 opportunities

Step 2: Select the Situations and Tasks

Like the VSSA, Trina plans to embed the VSSI within the context of his work experiences at the school. Trina, Sergio, and Sergio's parents have prioritized skills that will help Sergio obtain assistance when he needs materials and when he has completed his tasks. They also would like him to learn how to transition independently when he is given multiple tasks. Thus, his VSSI will include these three situations (materials needed, tasks completed, multiple tasks). To help promote generalization, Trina will include a variety of tasks and different reasons that Sergio might need materials for those tasks (e.g., because the materials are broken, missing, or of insufficient quantity). She also will include different task sequences in the multiple-task situation. She will use many of the same tasks that she included in the VSSA. They will include his regular tasks at the school store and cafeteria and some new tasks that Sergio is capable of completing when given clear instructions.

Step 3: Select the Interventions

Next, Trina considers the hierarchy of interventions to include in the VSSI. She begins by considering whether Sergio might benefit from spoken and written instructions alone. In her prior teaching experiences, she has found that Sergio typically needs more support to learn new skills. Trina then considers BST, the next intervention in the recommended hierarchy. In the past, Sergio has acquired some new skills after she briefly modeled the correct behavior and then had him practice it, although he has sometimes needed additional support following this initial training. Trina decides to begin the VSSI with BST for at least the first skill. She will introduce in-situ feedback, in-situ prompts, and in-situ reinforcement, if needed.

As discussed in Chapter 9, Trina knows that it is also important to consider the reinforcing consequences that Sergio receives for completing his vocational tasks. In the past, she has praised his work completion and has tried to be enthusiastic and supportive of his efforts. During the

VSSA, he completed his work when instructed, but he was heavily dependent on prompts to transition to new tasks and to obtain assistance with tasks that he couldn't complete. Thus, she now wonders if praise will be adequate to motivate Sergio to work during the VSSI. This motivation will be important when teaching him to ask for materials that he needs to complete his work, to notify his supervisor when he has completed his work, and to transition across multiple tasks. Ultimately, engaging in these behaviors (requesting assistance and transitioning across tasks) will enable Sergio to complete his work and, thus, receive reinforcement for doing so. Trina decides that Sergio would benefit from additional reinforcement for completing his work. To identify potential reinforcers for Sergio, Trina consults the list in Table 3.1 and also asks Sergio's caregivers to complete the reinforcer survey in Appendix A. After identifying a number of potential reinforcers, Trina conducts a preference assessment with Sergio using the instructions and data sheets in Appendix A. Results of this assessment suggest that Sergio really enjoys soft drinks, chips, and music. Her plan is to offer him a short (5 minute) break and a choice of these reinforcers whenever he completes a task or, in the case of the multiple-task situation, when he has completed a short sequence of assigned tasks.

Step 4: Develop the Intervention Plan

Based on her prior experience with Sergio, Trina believes that he would do best if she teaches one skill at a time. However, for the situations that involve seeking assistance from the supervisor, she will teach the two targets (seeks assistance and presses the relevant icon on the iPad) at the same time. Trina is now ready to start the VSSI plan for Sergio. She decides to begin the VSSI with the work-completed situation. As shown in Table 12.1, Trina drafts just the first four sessions as the plan will change depending on Sergio's performance.

Table 12.1 The First Four Sessions of Sergio's VSSI Plan

Session #	Target(s)	Intervention	Situation(s)	Task(s)	Materials
1	Seeks assistance; Presses icon	BST	Work Completed	Open boxes	5 boxes
2	Seeks assistance; Presses icon	BST	Work Completed	Sort materials	Various materials in 5 boxes
3	Seeks assistance; Presses icon	BST	Work Completed	Stock shelves	Various materials in 5 boxes
4	Seeks assistance; Presses icon	BST	Work Completed	Sweep	Broom; dustpan

Step 5: Establish a Plan for Monitoring and Interpreting Performance

Next, Trina establishes her system for collecting data and monitoring his performance during the VSSI. She will use the template version of the **Arranged Situations Data Sheet** to collect data on his performance during the three situations that will be included in his VSSI.

After each class period, she will graph his performance from each work session using the percentage-based version of the **VSSI Graphing Template**. For the work-completed and materials-needed situations, Trina will collapse the data collected for the two targeted responses (seeks assistance and presses icon) and plot the outcome on separate graphs for each situation. Thus, for each session, Trina will plot 0% if he does not engage in either behavior correctly, 50% if he engages in one of the two behaviors correctly, and 100% if he engages in both of the behaviors correctly. For transitioning independently across multiple (three) tasks, Trina will calculate the percentage of transitions that he completes independently in the session. With three tasks, Sergio will encounter just two transitions, so Trina will plot 0% if he doesn't transition independently across both transitions, 50% if he transitions independently for one of the two transitions, and 100% if he does so for both.

Step 6: Establish a Plan for Maintenance and Generalization

Even before starting the VSSI, Trina considers how she might ensure that Sergio's skills maintain over time and generalize to new work environments. After consulting Chapter 11, she develops the following plan:

Maintenance

If Sergio requires in-situ feedback, Trina will gradually fade out positive feedback for correct responses by providing feedback intermittently. She will begin by providing this feedback for every other correct response, then for every third correct response, and so forth, as long as he continues to respond correctly. She will use the same strategy to fade reinforcement if she ultimately includes it in any of the inventions. Finally, if he requires prompts, she will systematically delay her prompts over time.

Generalization

Trina will incorporate multiple exemplars into his training by (a) conducting the VSSI in both the school store and cafeteria, (b) recruiting several other teachers to occasionally serve as the supervisor, and (c) including a variety of tasks and materials. The cafeteria and school store already capitalize on the strategy to "incorporate common stimuli" because they are set up to resemble an actual retail store and restaurant where students may someday work.

However, before proceeding with the VSSI, Trina also considers whether Sergio is likely to receive effective, naturalistic reinforcement for engaging in these behaviors on the job. She answers the questions outlined in Chapter 11 and on the Identifying Natural Consequences Worksheet in Appendix A for each of his targeted behaviors. In terms of immediate consequences, all of the targeted responses will permit Sergio to complete his tasks and, thus, receive reinforcement for doing so, assuming that supervisors arrange effective reinforcement for task completion. With this in mind, Trina plans to recommend that Sergio receive highly preferred tangible reinforcers for completing tasks on any future job sites.

Step 7: Conduct Baseline and Begin Graphing

Trina examines the data she collected during the VSSA and determines that they are appropriate to use as her baseline for the VSSI. She graphs these baseline data, beginning with the work-completed situation. Because he never approached his supervisor and told her that he was finished during the VSSA, Trina just graphs the last four opportunities to do so from the assessment, as shown in Figure 12.1.

Step 8: Conduct the VSSI

Trina begins by using BST to teach Sergio to seek assistance and press the "finished" icon on his iPad when he has completed his work. Trina first works with Sergio in the school store. His regular duties during each class period are to open boxes, sort the merchandise, and stock shelves. To arrange efficient teaching sessions, Trina gathers a small amount of merchandise to use during the sessions. Trina first describes and models

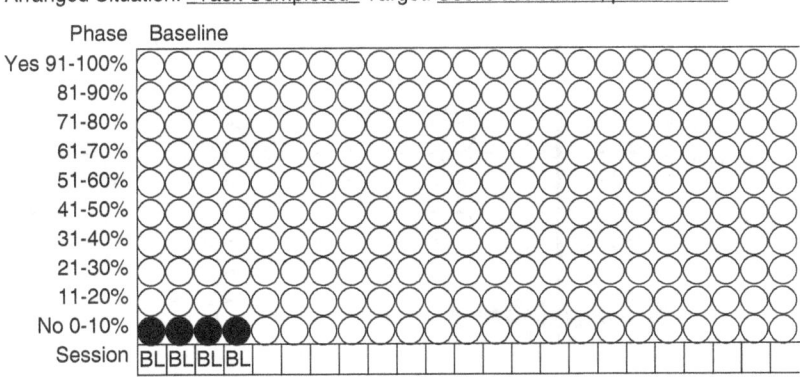

Figure 12.1 Example graph displaying Sergio's baseline data on responding appropriately during the work-completed situation.

the correct responses and then asks Sergio to practice. She instructs him to sort a small amount of merchandise and, when finished, to walk over to Trina and press the "finished" icon on his iPad. She also has Sergio practice by asking him to stock a small amount of merchandise on the shelves and to open a few boxes. She provides both positive and corrective feedback as he practices, using as much assistance as needed for Sergio to engage in the correct responses. Once Sergio has responded correctly three times, Trina has Sergio complete his regular duties at the school store while collecting data on the help-seeking behavior that Sergio has just practiced in the BST session.

Beginning with Session #1 of the VSSI plan, Trina instructs Sergio to open five boxes. As in the VSSA, she lets Sergio know that she will be working at a desk on the other side of the store and to let her know if he needs anything. She always waits at least 2 minutes after he completes his task to see if he will seek her assistance. She makes certain to provide a 5-minute break with his choice of reinforcer (soda, chips, music) for completing each task even if he does not seek her assistance.

Because Sergio does not engage in the correct responses when he finishes the first task (opening five boxes), she repeats the BST session the next time he is scheduled to work in the school store. This BST session is followed by Session #2 of the plan during which Trina asks Sergio to sort merchandise from five boxes. She continues to follow the plan because Sergio does not respond correctly following four sessions of BST, which included a session in the cafeteria (Session #4).

Trina's graph thus far is shown in Figure 12.2. Based on her intervention-change criterion, Trina now needs to introduce the next intervention in the hierarchy, in-situ feedback. She outlines the next four sessions of his VSSI plan, as shown in Table 12.2

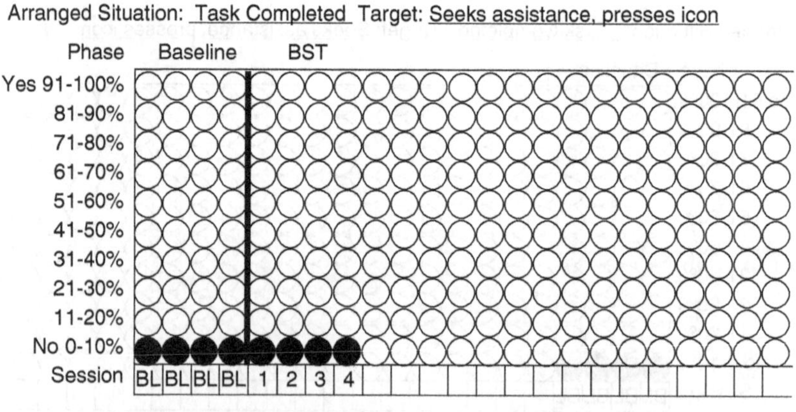

Arranged Situation: <u>Task Completed</u> Target: <u>Seeks assistance, presses icon</u>

Figure 12.2 Updated graph displaying Sergio's data on responding appropriately during the work-completed situation after receiving behavioral skills training (BST).

Table 12.2 Sessions 5–8 of Sergio's VSSI Plan

Session #	Target(s)	Intervention	Situation(s)	Task(s)	Materials
5	Seeks assistance; Presses icon	Feedback	Work Completed	Open boxes	5 boxes
6	Seeks assistance; Presses icon	Feedback	Work Completed	Sort materials	Various materials in 5 boxes
7	Seeks assistance; Presses icon	Feedback	Work Completed	Stock shelves	Various materials in 5 boxes
8	Seeks assistance; Presses icon	Feedback	Work Completed	Sweep	Broom; dustpan

As Sergio finishes each task, Trina waits 2 minutes to see if he will independently seek assistance. If Sergio responds correctly, Trina provides positive feedback by saying, "Nice job letting me know that you are done with your work!" If he does not, Trina provides corrective feedback by approaching Sergio and saying, "If you are done _____, you need to come find me and tell me using your iPad. Go ahead and show me." She then returns to her desk across the room and gives him an opportunity to practice one time.

Trina is pleased when Sergio begins to independently seek her assistance and press the "finished" icon on the iPad, starting with Session #7. She continues to add to her VSSI plan and to assess this skill until he meets the acquisition criterion of 100% responding across six consecutive opportunities. Her updated graph is shown in Figure 12.3

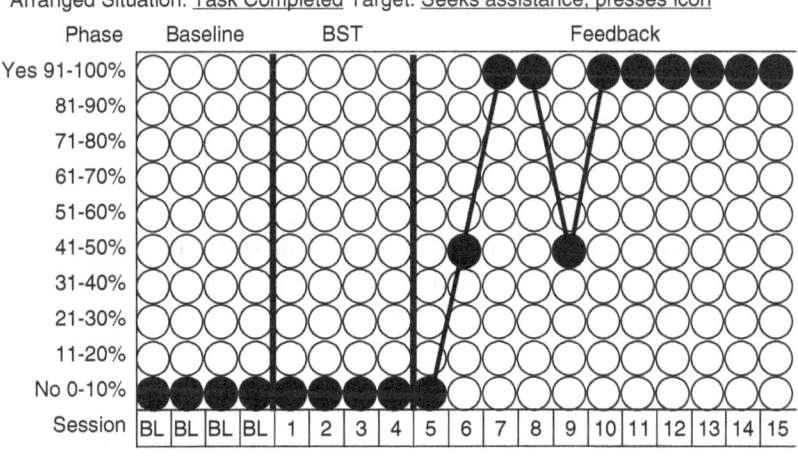

Figure 12.3 Updated graph displaying Sergio's data on responding appropriately during the work-completed situation after receiving in-situ feedback.

For her next step, Trina will begin to fade out the feedback and monitor maintenance of this target while introducing BST for the next target, requesting help when materials are needed. Because Sergio required BST plus in-situ feedback for the first skill and because Trina feels that this is a more complex situation, Trina decides to combine BST with in-situ feedback from the very first VSSI session. She will repeat BST at the start of each class period if Sergio required feedback during the previous class period. She will continue to arrange the materials-needed situation during work sessions until he meets the acquisition criterion or the intervention-change criteria.

To help stay organized, Trina outlines the next four sessions for the VSSI as shown in Table 12.3. She can easily combine the materials-needed and task-completed situations in each work session. Thus, in addition to his new skill, she will continue to monitor his performance in seeking her assistance and pressing the "finished" icon when he completes each task while she provides positive feedback intermittently according to the plan described previously.

Before starting the work sessions shown in Table 12.3, Trina conducts BST to introduce help-seeking in the materials-needed situation. Like her previous BST sessions, Trina gives Sergio a small amount of work to increase the efficiency of the practice; however, she ensures that he encounters either missing, broken, or insufficient amount of materials. Once Sergio responds correctly three times during these practice sessions, Trina has Sergio complete his regular duties while providing in-situ feedback if needed. She continues to collect data on his performance. Sergio meets the acquisition criterion (correct responding across six consecutive opportunities) after nine total sessions and continues to request help when he has completed his work during most sessions. Trina's updated graphs for both targets are displayed in Figure 12.4

Trina is now ready to introduce an intervention for Sergio's final targeted skill, transitioning independently across multiple tasks. Trina decides that the most efficient way to start the training for this particular skill is to omit the initial BST prior to his work sessions and provide in-situ feedback when she instructs him to complete three tasks in a specific sequence. To ensure that he continues to maintain the other two skills, Trina will occasionally arrange the materials-needed situation within the context of the multiple tasks and monitor whether he responds correctly when he completes his work. She will provide feedback intermittently for these skills. Table 12.4 displays a portion of the sessions in her updated VSSI plan.

Sergio does not show an increase in transitioning independently across multiple tasks after four opportunities, so he has met the intervention-change criterion. Trina had planned to introduce in-situ prompts next, and she considers what might be the most effective type(s) of prompts for Sergio and this skill. Visual prompts in the form of gestures, models, and pictures

Table 12.3 Sessions 16–19 of Sergio's VSSI Plan

Session #	Target(s)	Intervention(s)	Situation(s)	Task(s)	Materials
16	Seeks assistance; Presses icon	BST + Feedback; Intermittent Feedback	Materials Needed; Task Completed	Sweep area	Broom (dustpan missing)
17	Seeks assistance; Presses icon	BST + Feedback; Intermittent Feedback	Materials Needed; Task Completed	Wipe 20 chairs	Disinfecting wipes (remove all but four wipes)
18	Seeks assistance; Presses icon	BST + Feedback; Intermittent Feedback	Materials Needed; Task Completed	Wipe 10 tables	Disinfecting wipes (container missing)
19	Seeks assistance; Presses icon	BST + Feedback; Intermittent Feedback	Materials Needed; Task Completed	Mop area	Bucket; soap; mop (handle broken)

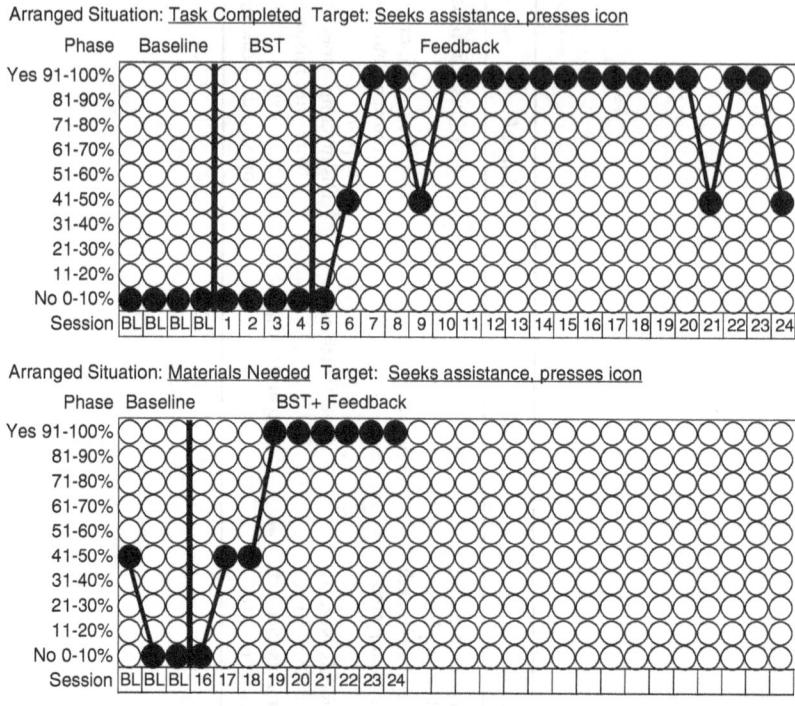

Figure 12.4 Updated graphs displaying Sergio's data on responding appropriately during the work-completed and materials-needed situations.

have been very effective for Sergio in the past. Trina also would like to reduce the likelihood of errors by initially presenting the prompt as soon as he has an opportunity to transition to the next task. Trina decides that she will gesture to the next task less than 1 minute after he completes the previous one and then gradually delay this prompt over time. However, Trina also considers the potential benefits of a picture prompt that could convey information about the assigned tasks and the desired task sequence. She decides to create a small board that would permit her to affix pictures of three assigned tasks arranged in the order of their desired completion. She will hand Sergio the board whenever she delivers her initial instruction. By creating pictures of all his tasks and using Velcro to affix them, Trina can prepare the picture board for each new work session.

Trina introduces these prompts while continuing to provide intermittent positive feedback for the previous skills. After the first work session, Sergio begins to transition independently across the tasks, and Trina fades out the gesture prompt. Before attempting to gradually fade out the picture prompt, she evaluates whether Sergio is still dependent on this prompt by omitting it from several work sessions. Trina is pleased to

Table 12.4 Sessions 25–27 of Sergio's VSSI

Session #	Target(s)	Intervention(s)	Situation(s)	Task(s)	Materials
25	Transitions; Seeks assistance; Presses icon	Feedback	Multiple Tasks; Task Completed	Sweep; Mop; Wipe 10 tables	Broom; dustpan; mop; bucket; soap; disinfecting wipes
26	Transitions; Seeks assistance; Presses icon	Feedback; Intermittent Feedback	Multiple Tasks; Task Completed	Open 5 boxes; Sort merchandise; Stock shelves	Boxes of merchandise
27	Transitions; Seeks assistance; Presses icon	Feedback; Intermittent Feedback; Intermittent Feedback	Multiple Tasks; Materials Needed; Task Completed	Clean shelves; Clean glass case; Clean cash register	Disinfecting wipes (container missing)

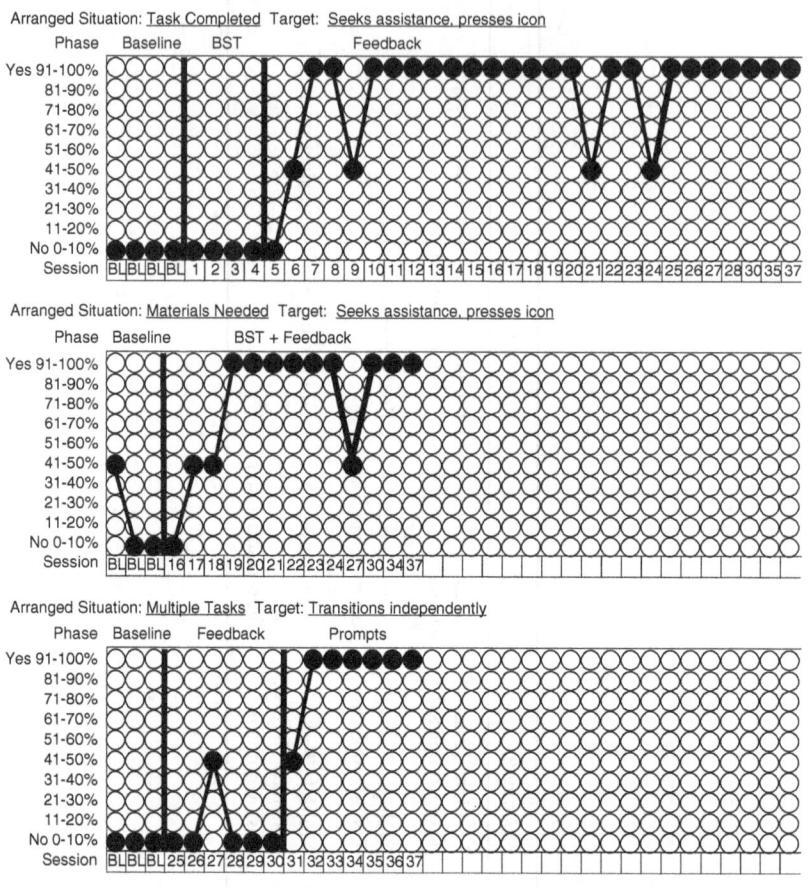

Figure 12.5 Updated graphs displaying all of Sergio's performance data during the VSSI.

observe Sergio continue to transition independently. Figure 12.5 displays all of Sergio's updated graphs.

Step 9: Assess Maintenance and Generalization

Now that Sergio has met all of his acquisition goals, Trina continues to arrange opportunities for him to engage in all three skills while monitoring his performance to determine if it will maintain. Referring back to his maintenance goals, she continues to monitor his performance to determine if it will maintain at the desired level across six weeks. She is careful to inspect her data frequently so that she can re-introduce intervention components if Sergio begins to struggle with any of the skills.

Referring back to his generalization goals, Trina arranges opportunities for Sergio to engage in the skills when he rotates to new work experiences at the school (e.g., assisting in the school library and front office). This permits her to evaluate his performance across new tasks, new task sequences, and new supervisors. If any of the skills do not successfully meet the generalization goal, Trina will reintroduce components of the intervention into the generalization context.

Case #2: Dayden

Dayden is a 25-year-old man with autism and mild intellectual disabilities who is receiving job placement and job coaching services through his local, state-funded vocational rehabilitation agency. His vocational counselor referred him to a local ABA center after he was terminated from two consecutive jobs. She would like Dayden to receive behavior intervention services so that he can be more successful at future job placements. Harlow, an instructor, conducted Dayden's VSSA at the ABA center.

The team considered the results of Dayden's assessment, along with his desired job placements and the reasons that he was terminated from his previous positions. Harlow explained the benefits of focusing on appropriate replacement behaviors for the inappropriate behaviors observed during the VSSA and at Dayden's prior jobs (arguing when given feedback and engaging in inappropriate conversation with others). With this in mind, Dayden and his team prioritized the following skills: (1) responding appropriately to feedback, (2) completing other work when the supervisor is not available to assist, and (3) engaging in appropriate conversation with customers and coworkers. The following describes how Harlow completes the steps needed to prepare for the VSSI, conduct the VSSI, and monitor Dayden's performance during the VSSI.

Step 1: Set Goals

Harlow's first step is to establish goals for the acquisition, maintenance, and generalization of the targeted skills. In collaboration with Dayden, he sets the following goals:

Acquisition Goals
- Target: Responding Appropriately to Feedback
     Goal: When Dayden is given corrective feedback, he will acknowledge the feedback ("say, I appreciate the input." "Thank you for letting me know."), ask clarifying questions if needed, confirm his understanding ("OK"), and then fix his mistakes across three consecutive opportunities.
- Target: Responding Appropriately When Supervisor is Unavailable
     Goal: When Dayden needs assistance but his supervisor is unavailable,

Dayden will immediately return to his work area, locate other tasks to complete, and work for at least 5 minutes before searching for his supervisor again across three consecutive opportunities.
- Target: Appropriate Conversation
  Goal: During simulated bagging sessions with customers or breaks with coworkers, Dayden will engage in appropriate conversation across six consecutive opportunities.

Maintenance and Generalization Goals
- Target: Responding Appropriately to Feedback
  Maintenance Goal: Dayden will respond appropriately to feedback on at least 90% of opportunities across two weeks.
  Generalization Goal: Dayden will respond appropriately to feedback across at least three different tasks, two different supervisors, and two different work locations.
- Target: Responding Appropriately When Supervisor is Unavailable
  Maintenance Goal: Dayden will respond appropriately when his supervisor is unavailable at least 90% of opportunities across two weeks.
  Generalization Goal: Dayden will respond appropriately when his supervisor is unavailable across at least two different supervisors and two different work locations.
- Target: Appropriate Conversation
  Maintenance Goal: During simulated bagging sessions with customers or breaks with coworkers, Dayden will engage in appropriate conversation on 80% of opportunities across two weeks.
  Generalization Goal: Sergio will respond correctly across at least two different customers, two different coworkers, and two different locations.

Harlow next selects a criterion for modifying the intervention (i.e., progressing to more intensive training) if Dayden does not make adequate progress during the VSSI. Harlow consults with Dayden's parents and also examines Dayden's prior education records. Based on this information, Harlow decides that he will modify the intervention for a target if Dayden does not show any improvement after three consecutive opportunities.

Intervention-Change Criteria
- No improvement across three consecutive opportunities

Step 2: Select the Situations and Tasks

Like the VSSA, Harlow will embed the VSSI within the context of simulated work at the ABA Center. Based on the prioritized skills, Harlow will need to arrange three situations that were also included in the VSSA (feedback provided, supervisor unavailable, breaks with coworkers). The supervisor-unavailable situation requires Dayden to need help from his supervisor during the VSSI. Thus, Harlow will ensure that Dayden does not know what to do next when he completes his assigned tasks and runs out or is missing materials during some of the work sessions. In order to target appropriate conversations with customers, Harlow decides to arrange a simulated-store situation during which either he or another staff person at the ABA center will pretend to be a customer who has just purchased merchandise and Dayden will be responsible for bagging the items. Along with the bagging task, Harlow will include many of the same tasks that he used during the VSSA when arranging situations that involve feedback and supervisor unavailability.

Step 3: Select the Interventions

Harlow next considers the hierarchy of interventions to include in the VSSI. He again reviews Dayden's education records and also asks Dayden's parents about the potential effectiveness of spoken and written instructions alone. Harlow learns that Dayden has modified his behavior when given rules and instructions in the past. Thus, he decides to start with spoken and written instructions. If this is not effective, he will introduce BST, followed by in-situ feedback, in-situ prompts, and in-situ reinforcement if needed.

Next, as discussed in Chapter 9, Harlow considers whether work completion itself is a reinforcer for Dayden, or if it might be beneficial to arrange reinforcers for completing assigned tasks during the VSSI. Because Dayden worked hard and seemed motivated to perform well on his tasks during the VSSA, Harlow decides to forgo this additional reinforcement for now.

Step 4: Develop the Intervention Plan

Based on information obtained from Dayden, his parents, and Dayden's prior education records, Harlow believes that Dayden could work simultaneously on the three targeted skills. An example of initial sessions that Harlow could implement during Dayden's first intervention appointment at the ABA center is shown in Table 12.5.

Step 5: Establish a Plan for Monitoring and Interpreting Performance

Harlow will use the template version of the **Arranged Situations Data Sheet** to collect data on his performance during the feedback and supervisor-unavailable situations. His third targeted skill, engaging in appropriate conversation with customers and peers, requires special consideration. During the VSSA, Harlow collected data on *inappropriate* conversation,

Table 12.5 Possible initial VSSI plan for Dayden's first appointment at the center

Session #	Target(s)	Intervention	Situation(s)	Task(s)	Materials
1	Responds to feedback	Spoken/Written Instructions	Feedback (Clear)	Stuff 15 envelopes	15 envelopes and letters
2	Works on other tasks	Spoken/Written Instructions	Missing Materials (napkins with supervisor); Supervisor Unavailable	Roll 10 sets of silverware	10 sets of silverware; 8 napkins
3	Engages in appropriate conversation	Spoken/Written Instructions	Simulated Store	Bag groceries	Variety of grocery items; 3 shopping bags Leisure materials
4	Engages in appropriate conversation	Spoken/Written Instructions	Break with Peer	N/A	
5	Works on other tasks	Spoken/Written Instructions	Task Completed; Supervisor Unavailable	Stock shelves	Variety of grocery items
6	Engages in appropriate conversation	Spoken/Written Instructions	Simulated Store	Bag office supplies	Variety of office supplies; 2 shopping bags
7	Responds to feedback	Spoken/Written Instructions	Feedback (Conflicting)	Clean 3 desks	Spray bottle, cloth
8	Engages in appropriate conversation	Spoken/Written Instructions	Break with Peer	N/A	Leisure materials

defined as asking personal questions or conveying information of a personal nature and initiating conversation about non-work related topics. However, Harlow plans to focus on teaching Dayden *appropriate* conversation topics to replace his inappropriate responses, an approach described in Chapter 1. To guide his intervention and data collection, Harlow establishes the following definitions of appropriate conversation with customers and coworkers after discussing possible options with Dayden:

Appropriate Conversation (Customers)

Greeting customers ("hello! How are today?"), responding to greetings ("I'm doing well"), thanking customers ("Thank you! Have a nice day!"), and inquiring about shopping satisfaction ("Did you find everything that you needed?") without asking personal questions, conveying information of a personal nature, or initiating a conversation about non-work topics.

Appropriate Conversation (Coworkers)

Conversing about work-related topics, hobbies, shared interests, and past activities without asking personal questions or conveying information of an inappropriately personal nature.

Harlow decides to collect data on appropriate conversation using the ***opportunity-based format*** of the **Additional Behaviors Data Sheet**. For each simulated customer interaction and each 5-minute break with a coworker, Harlow will score a "+" if Dayden's conversation meets the respective definitions above for the entire interaction. Thus, each encounter will be considered an opportunity.

After each session, Harlow will graph Dayden's performance using the percentage-based format of the **VSSI Graphing Template** found in Appendix B. For the feedback and supervisor-unavailable situations, Harlow will collapse the data collected for the responses targeted in each situation (i.e., calculate the percentage of responses implemented correctly) and plot the outcome on separate graphs for each situation. For appropriate conversation, Harlow will collect and plot the data separately for the simulated store and break situations. He will plot each opportunity using a "yes/no" format.

Step 6: Establish a Plan for Maintenance and Generalization

Next, Harlow considers which strategies he might use during the VSSI to ensure that Dayden's skills maintain until he starts his next job placement and to ensure that the skills generalize from the clinic to the actual work environment. After reviewing the strategies in Chapter 11, he outlines the following plan:

Maintenance

If Dayden is successful with any skills after receiving spoken and written instructions, Harlow will continue to monitor Dayden's performance periodically to determine if it will maintain. He will also ask Dayden if he is dependent on the written instructions and, if so, they will have a conversation about whether it might be helpful to retain this so that he can use it on the job site to help with both maintenance and generalization.

If Dayden requires in-situ feedback, Harlow will gradually fade out positive feedback for correct responses by providing feedback intermittently. He will begin by providing this feedback for every other correct response, then for every third correct response, and so forth, as long as Dayden continues to respond correctly. If Dayden requires prompts, Harlow will fade them depending on the modality he selects. He will use the same strategy to fade reinforcement if he ultimately includes it in any of the inventions.

Generalization

Harlow will incorporate multiple exemplars into his training by (a) including a variety of tasks, materials, and situations that require a supervisor's assistance (for supervisor unavailable), (b) recruiting several other staff to occasionally serve as the supervisor, simulated customer, and coworker, and (c) conducting the sessions in several different locations at the center. He will also arrange the work rooms so that they resemble actual store checkouts, break rooms, and offices to incorporate common stimuli by using actual groceries and office merchandise, real shopping bags, real stocking shelves, etc.

Next, Harlow meets with Dayden to discuss the potential naturalistic reinforcers that Dayden might receive for engaging in these behaviors on future job sites and, thus, help increase the likelihood that these skills will maintain over time. Together, they consider the immediate and delayed consequences of engaging in the targets or failing to engage in the targets, as suggested in Chapter 11. They used the Identifying Natural Consequences Worksheet in Appendix A to create the responses shown in Table 12.6.

Dayden assures Harlow that he wants to do well on his next job by completing his work correctly and remaining on task even when his supervisor is unavailable. He also very much enjoys when customers and coworkers respond to his social initiations, and he would like to make more friends. Dayden states that he wants to learn new skills that will help him achieve these goals. In light of these responses, Harlow believes that Dayden's targeted behaviors, which are intended to replace the inappropriate behaviors that resulted in his prior job termination, will receive naturalistic reinforcers on future job placements.

Table 12.6 Potential naturalistic consequences for Dayden's targeted skills

Target Behavior	*What are the immediate and delayed consequences of engaging in the behavior or failing to engage in the behavior?*
Respond appropriately to feedback	Immediate: Dayden is more likely to get the information he needs to complete his work correctly if he engages in the behavior. Delayed: Dayden may be more likely to retain his job if he consistently responds correctly.
Work on other tasks when supervisor is unavailable	Immediate: If Dayden does not begin additional tasks, the supervisor might correct him for taking an unauthorized break. Delayed: Dayden may be more likely to retain his job if he remains on task.
Engage in appropriate conversation with customers and coworkers	Immediate: Customers and coworkers are more likely to respond positively to Dayden's interactions. Delayed: Dayden may be more likely to retain his job if he engages in appropriate conversation with customers. He may be more likely to make friends with his coworkers.

Step 7: Conduct Baseline and Begin Graphing

Harlow considers whether the data he collected during the VSSA on these three skills would be appropriate to use as his baseline for the VSSI. Although the data collected on Dayden's performance when he received feedback or discovered that his supervisor was unavailable would provide an adequate baseline, Harlow recognized that the baseline for appropriate conversation would need special consideration. During the VSSA, Harlow collected data on inappropriate conversation using a frequency format and did not associate those data with any specific opportunities or situations. Further, he did not include a simulated store situation to evaluate this skill with customers. Harlow needs baseline data that are directly comparable to the data that he plans to collect during the VSSI.

To do so, Harlow now modifies his VSSI plan so that he can collect baseline data on Dayden's appropriate conversation during the simulated store and break situations. As illustrated in Table 12.7, Harlow will arrange those situations without introducing an intervention while collecting baseline data for several sessions.

Step 8: Conduct the VSSI

On the first day of the VSSI, Harlow meets with Dayden to provide spoken and written instructions on how to best respond to feedback. His

Table 12.7 Modifications to the first eight sessions of Dayden's VSSI plan

Session #	Target(s)	Intervention	Situation(s)	Task(s)	Materials
1	Responds to feedback	Spoken/Written Instructions	Feedback (Clear)	Stuff 15 envelopes	15 envelopes and letters
2	Works on other tasks	Spoken/Written Instructions	Missing Materials (napkins with supervisor); Supervisor Unavailable	Roll 10 sets of silverware	10 sets of silverware; 8 napkins
3	Engages in appropriate conversation	None (Baseline)	Simulated Store	Bag groceries	Variety of grocery items; 3 shopping bags
4	Engages in appropriate conversation	None (Baseline)	Break with Peer	N/A	Leisure materials
5	Works on other tasks	Spoken/Written Instructions	Task Completed; Supervisor Unavailable	Stock shelves	Variety of grocery items
6	Engages in appropriate conversation	None (Baseline)	Simulated Store	Bag office supplies	Variety of office supplies; 2 shopping bags
7	Responds to feedback	Spoken/Written Instructions	Feedback (Conflicting)	Clean 3 desks	Spray bottle, cloth
8	Engages in appropriate conversation	None (Baseline)	Break with Peer	N/A	Leisure materials

goal is to teach Dayden to engage in responses that would compete with arguing. Following the guidelines provided in Chapter 9, Harlow provides clear descriptions of the recommended responses, along with rationales and examples. He breaks the responses down into their component parts (e.g., acknowledge the feedback by saying, "Thank you for letting me know." or "I appreciate that!") and occasionally asks Dayden questions to assess his understanding. He also provides a written list of the responses similar to that shown in Table 9.1. Once Dayden indicates that he understands the instructions, Harlow implements Session #1 on his VSSI plan by instructing Dayden to return to the work room and stuff the envelopes on the desk. He reminds Dayden to keep the written instructions visible on his desk so that he can refer to them if needed. When Dayden indicates that he is finished, Harlow checks his work and tells him that he did not fold the letters correctly (provides feedback) to see if Dayden will engage in the instructed responses.

Harlow continues to follow his plan by introducing spoken and written instructions for the other targeted skill (working on other tasks when supervisor unavailable) while collecting baseline data on appropriate conversations. After graphing his baseline data for appropriate conversations with customers and coworkers, as shown in Figure 12.6, Harlow introduces spoken and written instructions for this skill. In doing so, he targets conversations with customers separately from those with coworkers, as they require somewhat different instructions and descriptions, as indicated by the definitions Harlow established in Step 5. He encourages Dayden to keep the written instructions handy during the simulated store and break situations.

As Harlow continues to implement the planned VSSI sessions, Dayden meets the acquisition criterion for working on other tasks when the supervisor is unavailable. However, he fails to make progress with the other skills, meeting the intervention-change criterion (no improvement across three consecutive opportunities). The graphed data for all skills are shown in Figure 12.7.

Harlow then implements BST for the unmastered skills, as this is the next intervention in the planned hierarchy. After reviewing the instructions for each skill, he provides opportunities for Dayden to practice the skills in roleplay by pretending to give him feedback about tasks and by having brief conversations in simulated bagging and break situations. Once Dayden responds correctly for several practice opportunities with each skill, Harlow resumes the arranged work situations for these skills. He also occasionally arranges the supervisor unavailable situation to evaluate maintenance and generalization of the associated target.

Dayden's correct response to feedback quickly meets the acquisition criterion following BST and he continues to work on other tasks when his supervisor is unavailable, but he does not make adequate progress on appropriate conversation. Although he has improved his interactions with

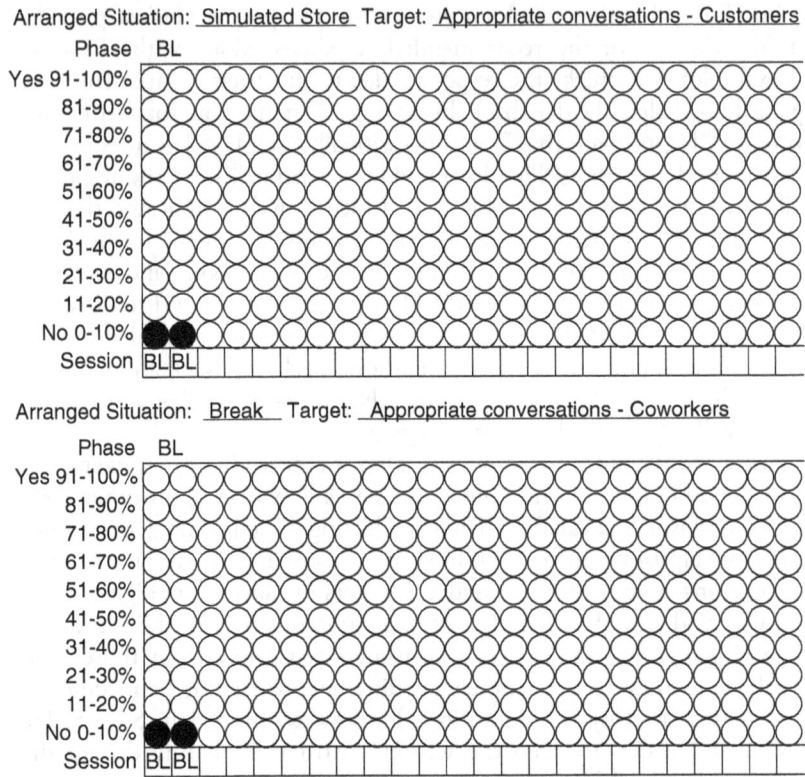

Figure 12.6 Graphs displaying Dayden's baseline data for appropriate conversations with customers and coworkers.

the simulated customers, Dayden continues to deviate from appropriate interactions with coworkers. His updated graphed data are shown in Figure 12.8.

Harlow now considers which intervention in the VSSI hierarchy would be most beneficial for Dayden and the targeted skill of appropriate conversation with coworkers. Although in-situ feedback is the next suggested intervention described in Chapter 9, Harlow speculates that this may be a relatively inefficient way to teach Dayden this skill. Further discussion with Dayden suggests that he is having difficulty thinking of appropriate conversation topics to discuss with coworkers in the moment and, thus, relies on a restricted set of topics, some of which are inappropriate (e.g., questions about intimate relationships or religion). In this case, Dayden may benefit most from a visual prompt that lists appropriate topics, comments, and questions that Dayden can reference when on breaks with coworkers. In collaboration with Dayden, Harlow

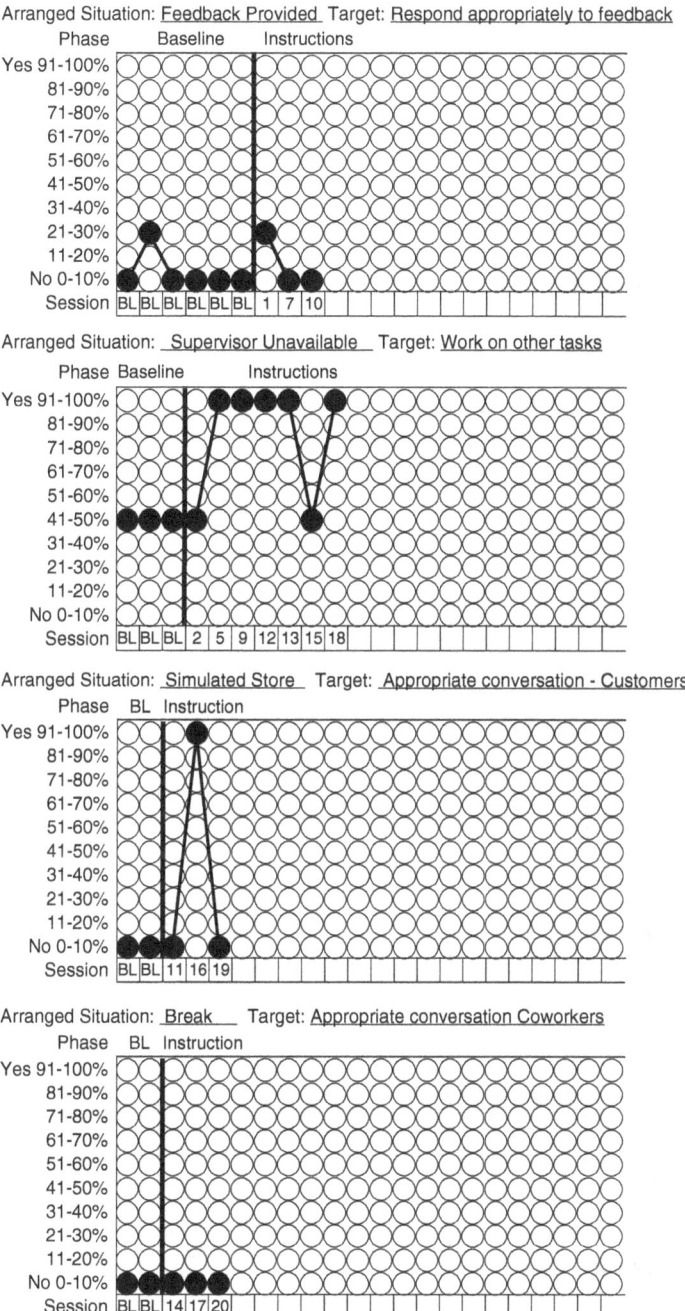

Figure 12.7 Graphs displaying data on Dayden's performance for all targeted skills after receiving spoken and written instructions.

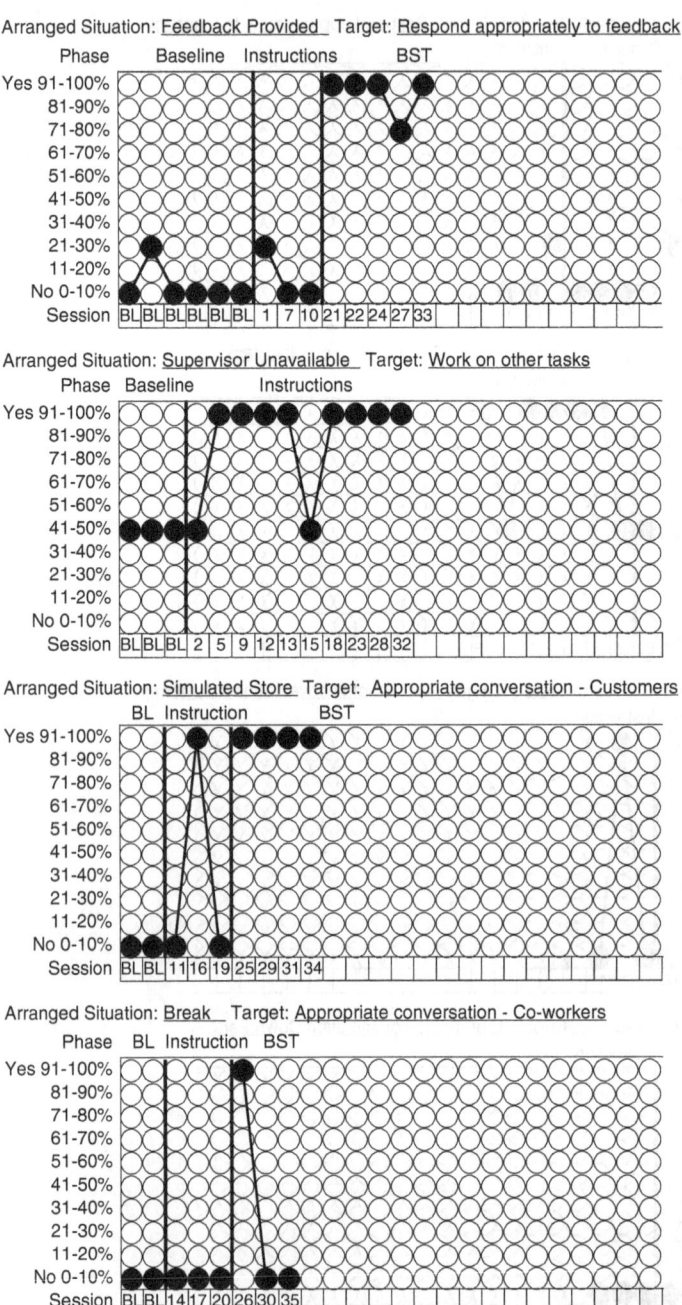

Figure 12.8 Updated graphs displaying data on Dayden's performance for all targeted skills during the VSSI.

Conversation Topics with Co-Workers
• What did you do last weekend/night/yesterday?
• What are your favorite sports/movies/video games?
• What do you like most about this job?
• How long have you worked here? Where else have you worked?
• Where did you go to school?

Figure 12.9 Dayden's visual prompt for engaging in appropriate conversation topics with conversation with coworkers.

creates the card shown in Figure 12.9. He also has Dayden take a picture of it so that he can reference it on his phone.

Harlow brainstorms with Dayden ways that he can easily access this card or its picture when interacting with coworkers. He then resumes the regular work sessions, using a plan that includes all arranged situations, while monitoring Dayden's progress on the remaining skill of engaging in appropriate conversation with coworkers, along with maintenance of the other skills. As shown in the updated graphs in Figure 12.10, the prompt is very helpful to Dayden. He also reports that he likes using it.

Step 9: Assess Maintenance and Generalization

Now that Dayden has met his acquisition goals, Harlow continues to arrange opportunities for him to engage in all his targeted skills while monitoring his performance to determine if it will maintain at the desired levels across two weeks, as indicated in his maintenance goals. In consideration of his generalization goals, Harlow also arranges opportunities for Dayden to engage in the skills when receiving feedback from another staff member at the center, to engage in conversation with a new coworker and simulated customer, and to complete tasks in a different location at the center (kitchen area). This permits Harlow to evaluate Dayden's performance across new people and locations before he informs Dayden's vocational counselor that Dayden is ready for a new job placement. If Dayden does not meet his generalization goals, Harlow will provide additional training.

Case #3: Anika

Anika is a 28-year-old woman with autism and moderate intellectual abilities who is receiving job training at a thrift shop for four hours each week with the assistance of a job coach provided by the VR office. Her job coach, Jaycee, would like to work on additional social and problem-solving

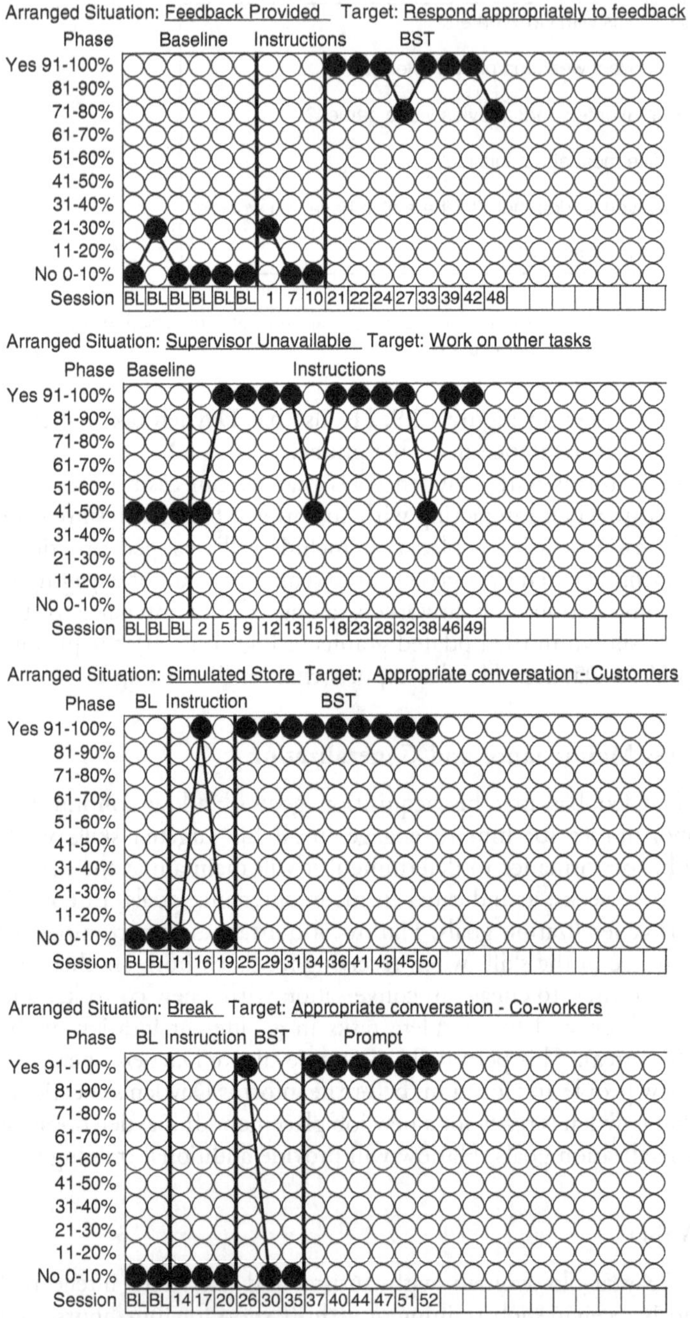
Arranged Situation: Feedback Provided Target: Respond appropriately to feedback
Phase Baseline Instructions BST
Yes 91-100%
81-90%
71-80%
61-70%
51-60%
41-50%
31-40%
21-30%
11-20%
No 0-10%
Session BL BL BL BL BL BL 1 7 10 21 22 24 27 33 39 42 48
Arranged Situation: Supervisor Unavailable Target: Work on other tasks
Phase Baseline Instructions
Session BL BL BL 2 5 9 12 13 15 18 23 28 32 38 46 49
Arranged Situation: Simulated Store Target: Appropriate conversation - Customers
Phase BL Instruction BST
Session BL BL 11 16 19 25 29 31 34 36 41 43 45 50
Arranged Situation: Break Target: Appropriate conversation - Co-workers
Phase BL Instruction BST Prompt
Session BL BL 14 17 20 26 30 35 37 40 44 47 51 52

Figure 12.10 Updated graphs displaying data on Dayden's performance for all targeted skills during the VSSI.

skills before recommending Anika for job placement services. Jaycee conducted Anika's VSSA at the thrift shop with the assistance of the shop supervisor.

Jaycee, Anika, her parents, and the shop supervisor considered which skills to prioritize for intervention in light of Anika's preferred job placements (office, movie theatre, animal shelter), the problematic behavior identified during the assessment (e.g., inappropriate requests), and Anika's personal goals. With these in mind, Anika and her team prioritized the following skills: (1) asking for help with tasks that Anika does not know how to complete, (2) recognizing when a supervisor needs help and offering assistance appropriately, (3) ensuring that Anika's brings everything that she needs to work (particularly, snacks and money), (4) responding appropriately when someone refuses a request, and (5) orienting towards others during conversational exchanges. The following describes how Jaycee prepares for the VSSI, conducts the VSSI, and monitors Anika's performance during the VSSI.

Step 1: Set Goals

Jaycee and Anika begin the process by establishing the following goals for the acquisition, maintenance, and generalization of the targeted skills.

Acquisition Goals
- Target: Responding Appropriately When Given Tasks She Does Not Know How To Complete:
  Goal: When given vague instructions or tasks not in her repertoire, Anika will seek her supervisor within 2 minutes of receiving the task and ask for help by saying, "Can you show me how"? "I need a model." "I don't know how to do this." "How would you like this done?" or similar statements across four consecutive opportunities.
- Target: Providing Unsolicited Help to Supervisor
  Goal: When her supervisor clearly needs assistance, Anika will offer to help by asking, "Can I help?" "Do you need any assistance?" or a similar question, provide the assistance for an adequate duration, and then return to her work within 1 minute of assisting across four consecutive opportunities.
- Target: Bringing Everything Needed to Work:
  Goal: Anika will bring at least one snack and $1.50 for the vending machine to work across four consecutive shifts.
- Target: Responding Appropriately to Refusals to Honor Requests
  Goal: When someone refuses to honor a request, Anika will say, "OK" in a calm tone and walk away across four consecutive opportunities.
- Target: Orienting
  Goal: When interacting with her supervisor (listening or speaking), Anika's face will be oriented towards the supervisor, except when

visually attending to relevant task materials (e.g., looking at task materials while the supervisor provides a model for completing the task) for at least 80% of the exchanges across three consecutive days.

Maintenance and Generalization Goals

- Target: Responding Appropriately When Given Tasks She Does Not Know How To Complete

  Maintenance Goal: Anika will respond appropriately when given vague instructions or tasks not in her repertoire at least 90% of opportunities across two weeks.

  Generalization Goal: Anika will respond appropriately when given vague instructions or tasks not in her repertoire across at least two different supervisors and two different work locations.

- Target: Providing Unsolicited Help to Supervisor

  Maintenance Goal: When her supervisor clearly needs assistance, Anika will respond appropriately on at least 70% of opportunities across two weeks.

  Generalization Goal: When her supervisor clearly needs assistance, Anika will respond appropriately across at least three different types of situations, two different supervisors, and two different locations.

- Target: Bringing Everything Needed to Work:

  Maintenance Goal: Anika will bring at least one snack and $1.50 for the vending machine to at least 80% of her work shifts across one month.

  Generalization Goal: Anika will bring necessary food and money to a new job setting (to be assessed when Anika starts a new job.)

- Target: Responding Appropriately to Refusals to Honor Requests

  Maintenance Goal: When someone refuses to honor her request, Anika will say, "OK" in a calm tone and walk away on at least 90% of opportunities across two weeks.

  Generalization Goal: When someone refuses to honor her request, Anika will respond appropriately across at least two different coworkers.

- Target: Orienting

  Maintenance Goal: When interacting with her supervisor (listening or speaking), Anika's face will be oriented towards the supervisor on at least 70% of opportunities across two weeks.

  Generalization Goal: Anika will orient towards her supervisor when listening or speaking across at least two different supervisors and two different locations.

Jaycee next selects a criterion for modifying the intervention (i.e., progressing to more intensive training) if Anika does not make adequate progress during the VSSI. Based on her prior experiences with Anika at the thrift shop, Jaycee decides that she will modify the intervention for a target if Anika does not show any improvement after three consecutive opportunities, with the exception of orienting. She will modify the intervention for orienting if Anika does not show any improvement for three consecutive work shifts or fails to meet the acquisition criterion after 10 work shifts. She included this latter criterion because Anika said that it may be quite difficult for her to learn to orient consistently. Thus, Anika might show some improvement but still fail to acquire the skill in a timely manner. By including a criterion based on the total number of shifts without meeting the criterion, Jaycee hopes to increase the efficiency of the VSSI. The following summarizes her criteria:

Intervention-Change Criteria
* No improvement across three consecutive opportunities (for all but orienting)
* No improvement across three consecutive work shifts (for orienting only)
* Failure to meet the acquisition goal after 10 work shifts (for orienting only)

Step 2: Select the Situations and Tasks

Jaycee will continue to work with Anika at the thrift shop with the assistance of the shop supervisor. Based on the prioritized skills, Jaycee will need to arrange two situations that she also included in the VSSA (vague instructions or task not in repertoire, supervisor in need of assistance). For the supervisor-in-need-of-assistance situation, Jaycee and the shop supervisor will continue to spill items or attempt to lift/move heavy boxes near Anika while she is working to provide opportunities for her to offer unsolicited help to others. She will embed the VSSI within Anika's responsibilities at the thrift shop but also include some new tasks to arrange the vague-instructions and task-not-in-repertoire situations. Opportunities for her to bring snacks and money to work will occur for each shift at the shop.

To set up opportunities for her to respond appropriately when coworkers refuse her requests, Jaycee will ask all shop staff to no longer honor Anika's requests for food or money. Thus, opportunities for her to respond appropriately in this situation should occur every time she asks a coworker for either food or money. Finally, opportunities for Anika to orient toward her supervisor will occur whenever Anika initiates interactions with a supervisor or whenever they deliver instructions or feedback to Anika.

Step 3: Select the Interventions

Jaycee next considers the hierarchy of interventions to include in the VSSI. Based on her experiences working with Anika, she does not think that spoken and written instructions alone are likely to be sufficient in teaching these particular skills. However, Anika has responded well to BST in the past. Thus, Jaycee will begin with BST, followed by in-situ feedback, in-situ prompts, and in-situ reinforcement if needed.

However, one targeted skill requires special consideration because it must be performed outside of the work setting. Interventions to ensure that Anika brings her snack and money to work must be arranged in her home before she starts her work shift. Because Jaycee only works with Anika at the shop, she considers the types of interventions that Anika's mother could effectively employ at home. However, she would like Anika to be as independent as possible; thus, she considers the potential of helping Anika to use technology-based prompts, such as cell phone reminders or alarms. Jaycee decides that she will start with these types of prompts and add in-situ reinforcement if needed. She will ask Jaycee's mother to ensure that snacks and money are available to Anika at home.

Next, as discussed in Chapter 9, Jaycee considers whether work completion itself is a reinforcer for Anika, or if it might be beneficial to arrange reinforcers for completing new or difficult assigned tasks during the VSSI. Anika typically works hard and seems to have a strong desire to please others. Thus, Jaycee decides to forgo this additional reinforcement for now but will remember to acknowledge her efforts to complete her work.

Step 4: Develop the Intervention Plan

Jaycee believes that Anika might struggle if she attempts to work simultaneously on all five targeted skills. Because Anika expressed a great deal of excitement about learning to provide unsolicited help to her supervisor, Jaycee would like to prioritize this skill and teach it simultaneously with two other targets. She decides to target asking for help with tasks, given the importance of this skill, along with bringing snacks and money to work. If Anika is successful in acquiring the latter skill, she will be less likely to request food and money from coworkers and, thus, less likely to encounter refusals. Once Anika acquires these skills, Jaycee will introduce intervention for the remaining two skills.

Jaycee outlines her initial sessions with the two skills that will be targeted within the work setting, as shown in Table 12.8. For the home-based target, Jaycee will meet with Anika to discuss potential technology-based prompts and help her set them up on her cell phone. Then, she will check with her at the start of each work shift to see if she remembered her snacks and money.

Table 12.8 First six work sessions of Anika's VSSI plan

Session #	Target(s)	Intervention	Situation(s)	Task(s)	Materials
1	Provide unsolicited help	BST	Supervisor Needs Assistance (moves heavy boxes from unloading area)	Sort donations	5 boxes
2	Ask for help	BST	Vague Instructions	Organize books	20 books
3	Ask for help	BST	Task Not In Repertoire	Create spreadsheet	Laptop; inventory list
4	Provide unsolicited help	BST	Supervisor Needs Assistance (spills a large bucket of blocks nearby)	Mop floor	Mop; bucket; soap
5	Ask for help	BST	Vague Instructions	Stock shelves	Variety of merchandise
6	Provide unsolicited help	BST	Supervisor Needs Assistance (drops stack of papers)	File	File box; 20 letters

Step 5: Establish a Plan for Monitoring and Interpreting Performance

Jaycee will use the template version of the ***Arranged Situations Data Sheet*** to collect data on Anika's performance during vague-instructions, task-not-in-repertoire, and supervisor-needs-assistance situations. For the remaining targets (bringing snacks and money to work, responding appropriately to refusals, orienting), Jaycee will collect data using the ***opportunity-based format*** of the ***Additional Behaviors Data Sheet***. For each work shift, Jaycee will record whether Anika brought her snacks and money that day. Each time she learns that Anika has asked a coworker for food or money, she will record whether Anika responded appropriately to the refusal. Finally, each time that Anika and her supervisor converse, Jaycee will record whether or not Anika oriented towards the supervisor (face directed towards the supervisor, except when visually attending to relevant task materials) for the duration of the interaction.

After each session, Jaycee will graph Anika's performance using the percentage-based version of the ***VSSI Graphing Template***. For vague-instructions, task-not-in-repertoire, and supervisor-needs-assistance situations, Jaycee will collapse the data collected for the responses targeted in each situation (i.e., calculate the percentage of responses implemented correctly) and plot the outcome on separate graphs for each situation. For each work shift, she will plot a "yes" or "no" to indicate whether she brought her snacks and money. Because Anika is unlikely to have an opportunity to respond to refusals more than once per work shift (based on the data from the VSSA [i.e., her baseline]), Jaycee also will plot a "yes" or "no" for each opportunity to respond. For orienting, Jaycee will calculate the number of interactions with correct orienting and divide this number by the total number of opportunities scored to determine the percentage of opportunities with correct orienting.

Step 6: Establish a Plan for Maintenance and Generalization

Next, Jaycee considers how she might help Anika maintain the skills over time, as well as increase the likelihood that the skills Anika learns at the thrift shop will transfer to her future new job placements. The following outlines her plan:

Maintenance

For any skill(s) that Anika acquires with BST, Jaycee will continue to monitor her performance periodically to determine if the skill(s) maintain. If Anika requires in-situ feedback or reinforcement, Jaycee will gradually fade out positive feedback and reinforcement by providing these consequences intermittently. She will begin by providing consequences for every other correct response, then for every third correct response, and so forth, as long as she continues to respond correctly. If Anika requires prompts, she will fade them in ways that will be determined by the prompt modalities. However, Jaycee will ask Anika if she wants to retain or fade the technology-based prompt if she finds it effective for managing her own behavior.

Generalization

Jaycee will incorporate multiple exemplars into Anika's training by (a) using a variety of tasks and materials that require the supervisor's assistance to complete, (b) arranging different reasons that the supervisor might need assistance, (c) recruiting other staff to occasionally serve as the supervisor, and (d) conducting work sessions in several different locations at the thrift shop.

As part of her maintenance plan, Jaycee also meets with Anika to discuss possible naturalistic reinforcers that might help maintain Anika's skills on future job sites. Together, they use the Identifying Natural Consequences Worksheet in Appendix A to list possible immediate and delayed consequences of engaging in each target or failing to engage in each target. As they discuss the possible consequences, shown in Table 12.9, Anika confirms that she values the potential immediate or

Table 12.9 Potential naturalistic consequences for Anika's targeted skills

Target Behavior	What are the immediate and delayed consequences of engaging in the behavior or failing to engage in the behavior?
Ask for help with tasks	Immediate: Anika will get the information she needs to complete her work correctly. Delayed: Anika will be considered a valuable employee because she completes her work correctly.
Offer unsolicited assistance	Immediate: Anika will receive the gratitude of others. Delayed: Anika will build good social relations.
Bring everything needed to work	Immediate: Anika will be able to get snacks when hungry. Delayed: None
Respond appropriately to refusals	Immediate: If Anika responds inappropriately, her coworkers may become angry. Delayed: Anika may build good social relations if she responds appropriately. If not, her coworkers may begin to avoid her.
Orient during interactions	Immediate: If Anika does not orient, her conversation partner may think that she is not interested and may terminate the interaction. Delayed: Anika may build good social relations by orienting consistently. If she does not orient consistently, people may avoid interacting with her because she may not seem interested in doing so.

delayed reinforcers that may occur if she engages in the targeted skills at future job sites.

Step 7: Conduct Baseline and Begin Graphing

Jaycee determines that the data she collected on four of the five targeted responses during the VSSA would be appropriate to use as her baseline for the VSSI. However, she has not yet collected pre-intervention (i.e., baseline) data on the target of bringing snacks and money to work. Thus, before starting the VSSI, she collects these data across four consecutive work shifts. Examples of her graphs with baseline data (for providing unsolicited help and bringing snacks and money to work) are shown in Figure 12.11.

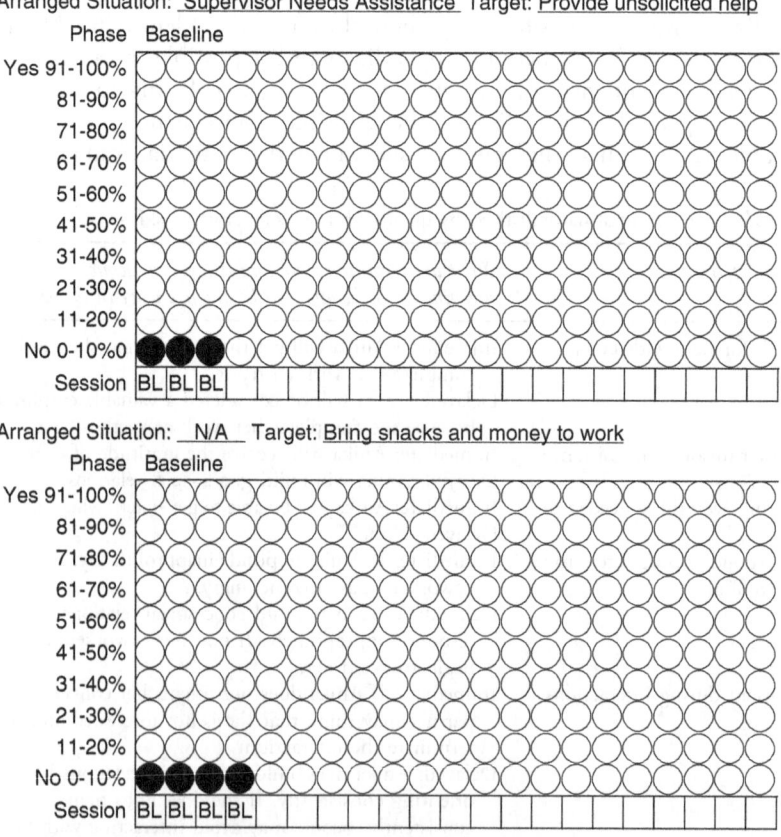

Figure 12.11 Graphs displaying Anika's baseline data on providing unsolicited help and bringing snacks and money to work.

Step 8: Conduct the VSSI

On the first day of the VSSI, Jaycee meets with Anika at the start of her shift at the thrift shop. She first helps Anika set up a recurring alarm on her cell phone, which Anika selected as the technology-based prompt to help remind her to pack a snack and money in her work bag about one hour prior to each shift. Anika practices setting the alarm in case she needs to modify it in the future.

Jaycee then implements BST for the targeted skills of providing unsolicited assistance and asking for help. She begins with the target of providing unsolicited assistance, as indicated in her initial VSSI plan. After describing the benefits of helping her supervisor and the various situations that would be appropriate to offer help, Jaycee models the correct responses. She then roleplays with Anika by pretending to need help in various ways. When Anika responds correctly for several practice opportunities, Jaycee introduces BST for the second targeted skill, asking for help. Jaycee again combines instructions, modeling, and practice, continuing to role play until Anika responds correctly for several consecutive roleplays.

Jaycee then asks Anika to begin her work shift as usual, assigning her the tasks and arranging the situations planned for the first six sessions of the day, as shown in Table 12.8. The thrift shop supervisor and Jaycee take turns providing Anika with her work assignments or acting as though they need assistance (e.g., by attempting to move a number of heavy boxes near Anika's work area; spilling items).

As the VSSI continues, Anika quickly meets the acquisition goal for the target of offering unsolicited assistance and maintains her performance over time. Anika also finds the phone alerts helpful for remembering to bring her snacks and money to work. In fact, she only fails to bring her snack one day since the start of this intervention. On that day, Anika explains that she had run out of her preferred snacks at home.

Although asking for help improves somewhat, she does not meet her goal for this target due to the variability in her performance. As indicated by the graph in Figure 12.12 for this skill, Anika either emits none or both responses correctly. Jaycee examines her data sheets and notes that Anika always responded correctly when given a task not in her repertoire but not when given vague instructions. After Anika meets the intervention-change criterion by showing no improvement for three consecutive opportunities, Jaycee decides that Anika needs more support to ask for help in this situation.

Thus, Jaycee begins to provide in-situ feedback to help Anika meet her goal for this target. When Jaycee or the shop supervisor give Anika vague instructions about a new task, they wait to see if Anika will ask for help or clarification. They then praise Anika for engaging in correct responses (e.g., "Nice job asking me how to organize these items!") or tell her what

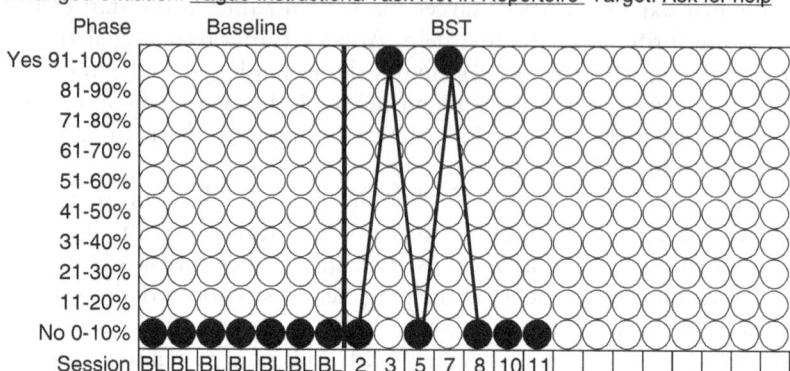

Figure 12.12 Graph displaying Anika's data on correctly asking for help after she received behavioral skills training (BST) for this skill.

she should have done differently (e.g., "You should have asked me to show you how to do this new task because I didn't tell you how."). Nonetheless, Anika continues to struggle with this target, again meeting the criterion to modify the intervention.

Next, Jaycee evaluates the effectiveness of in-situ prompts by giving Anika spoken reminders at the beginning of her work shifts ("Don't forget to ask for help if I give you a new task and don't show or tell you how to do it!") and a textual prompt that lists the desired responses, as illustrated in Figure 12.13. She includes multiple things that Anika could say when asking for help (e.g., "Can you should me how? "I need a model") on the textual prompt. However, Anika still has difficulty with this skill, and Jaycee notices that she never references the textual prompt.

Jaycee next considers introducing in-situ tangible reinforcement. Jaycee provides Anika with a list of various reinforcers that she could potentially earn for "remembering to ask for help" and invites her to choose her favorite ones. Among the potential items is monetary

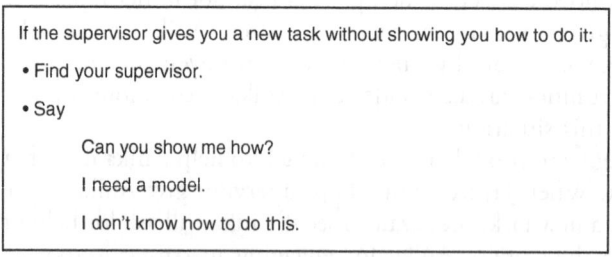

Figure 12.13 Visual prompt for Anika's skill of asking for help.

reinforcement because she knows that Anika is highly motivated to earn spending money. Anika asks to receive $.25 every time she asks for help when needed.

Jaycee continues the VSSI at the thrift shop, providing feedback, praise, and monetary reinforcement when Anika correctly asks for help. Jaycee also continues to monitor the maintenance of Anika's previously acquired skills. Anika, who is delighted to receive the monetary reinforcement, consistently asks for help when she receives a task that she does not know how to do, quickly meeting the acquisition goal. Jaycee's updated graph for this skill is shown in Figure 12.14.

Now that Anika has acquired her first three skills, Jaycee's next step is to introduce BST for the remaining skills (responding appropriately to refusals and orienting). However, because Anika is now successfully re-membering to bring her snacks and money to work, she has not requested these items from coworkers. At this point, Jaycee decides to prioritize orienting while periodically arranging opportunities to monitor the previously acquired skills and fading in-situ reinforcement as part of the maintenance plan. Table 12.10 shows an example of how Jaycee arranged these sessions within her VSSI plan. Once Jaycee introduces BST for orienting, she can begin to collect data on this behavior when opportu-nities arise in each work session (beginning with Session #26).

As Jaycee continues to implement the planned VSSI sessions, Anika has difficulty orienting during interactions with her supervisor but maintains her performance with the previously mastered ones. Anika repeatedly states that orienting is quite challenging for her. Thus, before proceeding any further, Jaycee asks Anika if she would still like to target this skill. Because Anika again assures Jaycee that she would like to learn how to "look at people when we talk," Jaycee considers what might be the most appropriate intervention for this skill.

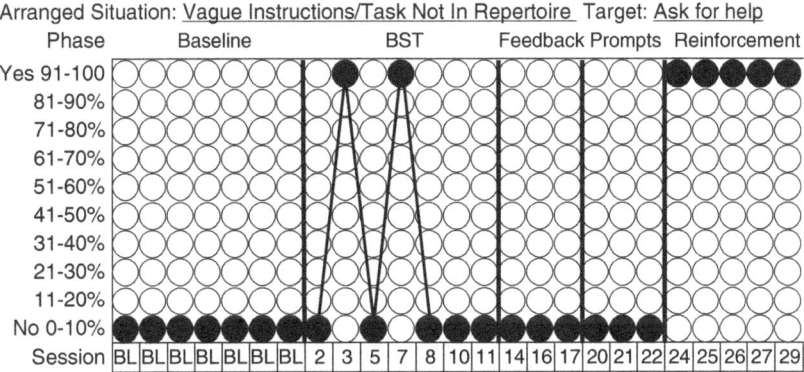

Figure 12.14 Updated graph displaying Anika's data on correctly asking for help during the VSSI.

Table 12.10 Sessions 26–30 of Anika's VSSI Plan

Session #	Target(s)	Intervention(s)	Situation(s)	Task(s)	Materials
26	Ask for help; Orient	Intermittent reinforcement; BST	Vague Instructions	Organize files	20 files
27	Ask for help; Orient	Intermittent reinforcement; BST	Task Not In Repertoire	Create graph	Data, computer
28	Provide unsolicited help; Orient	N/A; BST	Supervisor in Need of Assistance (drops a large stack of pencils that scatter)	Mop floor	Mop; bucket; soap
29	Ask for help; Orient	Intermittent reinforcement; BST	Vague Instructions	Stock shelves	Variety of merchandise
30	Orient	BST	N/A	File	File box; 20 letters

The remaining interventions in the VSSI hierarchy are in-situ feed-back, prompts, and reinforcement. It might be somewhat awkward to deliver in-situ feedback during ongoing social exchanges, so Jaycee next considers potential in-situ prompts that might work well. Jaycee briefly considers showing Anika a visual prompt (e.g., a card with a picture of a face oriented forward), but hesitates because Anika did not find a visual prompt helpful when learning to ask for help. Because Anika responded so well to monetary reinforcement, Jaycee decides to introduce this same reinforcer for orienting. Anika agrees that she might find this type of intervention helpful. To implement this intervention, Jaycee or the thrift shop supervisor provide the monetary reinforcer at the end of interactions if Anika remained oriented during the entire exchange.

As shown in Figure 12.15, Anika's performance rapidly improves once she starts to receive tangible reinforcement for this skill. She meets the acquisition criterion after nine work shifts (Session #39 on the graph in Figure 12.15) by orienting during at least 80% of the exchanges across three consecutive days.

Step 9: Assess Maintenance and Generalization

Anika has now met her acquisition goals for four targeted skills and has demonstrated maintenance of the first three targeted skills across at least two consecutive weeks (her maintenance goal). To fade the monetary reinforcement for requesting help and orienting, Jayce and the thrift shop supervisor begin to provide the monetary reinforcement intermittently. As indicated in the maintenance plan, they start providing $.25 for every other correct response, then for every third correct response, and so forth, as long

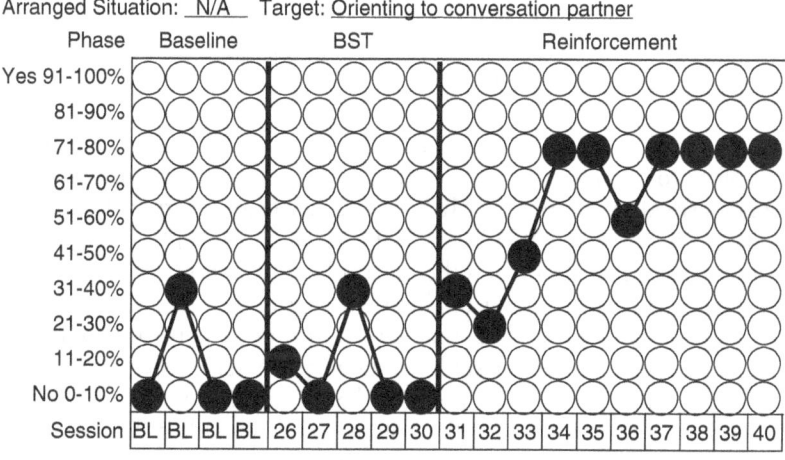

Figure 12.15 Graph displaying Anika's data on orienting during the VSSI.

as Anika continues to respond correctly. However, they continue to provide praise for correct responses. Once monetary reinforcement has been faded to every fifth correct response, Jaycee tells Anika that she will now just receive $1.00 at the end of each shift for "working hard." The money is not contingent on any particular level of performance. Rather than just eliminating the monetary reinforcer completely, Jaycee believes that this step will help her further fade the monetary reinforcer. Jaycee then begins to fade the praise in a similar manner while ensuring that Anika's behavior maintains.

For the final portion of her VSSI, Jaycee continues to arrange opportunities for Anika to engage in all skills to ensure that they maintain at the desired levels while she gradually fades the in-situ reinforcement and feedback for the targeted skills that required more than just BST. Jaycee does not develop a plan for fading the technology-based prompt because Anika stated that she prefers to keep using her cell phone alarm to remember to bring her snacks and money to work.

To help increase the likelihood of generalization, Jaycee also arranges opportunities for Anika to ask for help, provide unsolicited assistance, and to orient during interactions while another thrift shop employee must fill in for the shop supervisor and while Anika completes tasks in two new locations at the shop (the bathroom and employee breakroom). If Anika does not meet his generalization goals, Jaycee will provide additional training.

Case #4: Michelle

Michelle is a 19-year-old woman with autism, ADHD, and mild cognitive impairment who has no work or volunteer experience. Michelle lives with her parents in a rural area where there are no vocational rehabilitation services nearby. Michelle and her family requested telehealth services from their state vocational rehabilitation agency to help prepare Michelle for competitive employment. Bella, a job coach who works with an organization in their state, agreed to provide services via a videoconferencing platform. She conducted a VSSA via Zoom™ with the assistance of Michelle's mother. The vocational rehabilitation agency has now authorized 5 hours of intervention services. Based on the family's availability, Bella plans to conduct the VSSI during weekly 1-hour appointments.

As described in Chapter 7, Michelle and her team prioritized two skills based on results of the VSSA, Michelle's preferred job placement (small retail or department store), and the practical constraints of remote services. The skills include (1) asking for help with tasks that Michelle does not know how to complete and (2) making confirming statements when given task instructions. The latter skill was targeted to serve as a replacement behavior for complaints and protests that Michelle sometimes emitted when given task instructions. The following sections describe how Bella prepares for the VSSI, conducts the VSSI, and monitors Michelle's performance during the VSSI while providing remote services.

Step 1: Set Goals

Bella and Michelle first discuss potential goals for the acquisition, maintenance, and generalization of the targeted skills while considering the time-limited nature of the services (i.e., a total of 5 hours). Working together, they also identify appropriate statements that Michelle could make to request help and confirm understanding. Bella plans to have a coworker from her company serve as the supervisor during one of the appointments to evaluate the generalization goal. Together, Bella and Michelle draft the following goals:

Acquisition Goals
- Target: Responding Appropriately When Given Tasks You Do Not Know How To Complete:

    Goal: When given a new task without clear instructions, Michelle will call out for Bella within two minutes of receiving the task and ask for help by saying things like, "Can you show me how"? "I need a model." "How would you like this done?" or similar statements across four consecutive opportunities.
- Target: Confirm Understanding of Task Instructions:

    Goal: When given instructions to complete or to re-do a task (including corrections to her work), Michelle will confirm her understanding by saying "OK." "Will do." "Consider it done." "I will <repeat instruction>," or similar statement *without complaining or protesting* across eight consecutive opportunities.

Maintenance and Generalization Goals
- Target: Responding Appropriately When Given Tasks You Do Not Know How To Complete

    Maintenance Goal: Michelle will respond appropriately when given vague instructions on at least 100% of opportunities across three appointments.

    Generalization Goal: Michelle will respond appropriately when given vague instructions across at least two different supervisors.
- Target: Confirm Understanding of Task Instructions:

    Maintenance Goal: Michelle will confirm her understanding without complaining or protesting on at least 100% of opportunities across three appointments.

    Generalization Goal: Michelle will respond appropriately when given instructions across at least two different supervisors.

Bella next selects a criterion for modifying the intervention (i.e., progressing to more intensive training) if Michelle does not make adequate progress during the VSSI. Given the time-limited nature of her services,

Bella decides that she will modify the intervention for a target if Michelle does not show any improvement after two consecutive opportunities.

Intervention-Change Criteria
• No improvement across two consecutive opportunities

Step 2: Select the Situations and Tasks

Bella will continue to assign tasks and arrange situations remotely as she did for Michelle during the VSSA. Michelle's main work area will be the kitchen table. Prior to each appointment, Bella will send Michelle's mother a list of the necessary task materials so that she can make them accessible to Michelle on a nearby counter at the start of the appointment. Using the chat feature of Zoom™, Bella will send Michelle links to any materials needed for computer-related tasks, and she will instruct Michelle to share her screen so that Bella can view her work.

For her first target (asking for help), Bella will need to arrange the vague-instructions situation using tasks that she has never included in her sessions with Michelle. Opportunities to make confirming statements, her second target, will occur whenever Michelle receives any task instructions or feedback to change her work. Thus, Bella plans to assign a variety of tasks and to sometimes ask Michelle to correct or change her work.

Step 3: Select the Interventions

Bella next considers the hierarchy of interventions to include in the VSSI. Based on her review of Michelle's school records and information provided by Michelle's mother, Bella thinks that Michelle might acquire one or both responses with spoken and written instructions alone. This intervention might be particularly helpful if Bella teaches Michelle how to employ the written instructions as prompts while on the job. If these are not sufficient, Bella will introduce BST, followed by in-situ feedback, in-situ prompts, and in-situ reinforcement if needed. Based on Michelle's performance during the VSSA and her strongly expressed desire to start working, Bella suspects work completion itself is a reinforcer for Michelle. Thus, Bella will not provide additional reinforcement for task completion. However, she will deliver praise when Michelle completes her work correctly, particularly after she has successfully asked for instructions on how to do so.

Step 4: Develop the Intervention Plan

Bella and Michelle agree that she should work on both targets simultaneously, given the abbreviated nature of the VSSI and Michelle's likely success with an intervention for these two targets. Bella drafts the plan for the first appointment, as shown in Table 12.11. Because her intervention-change

Table 12.11 Sessions planned for Michelle's first VSSI appointment

Session #	Target(s)	Intervention	Situation(s)	Task(s)	Materials
1	Confirm understanding	Spoken/Written Instructions	N/A	Staple	10 sets of papers; stapler with 10 staples
2	Ask for help; Confirm understanding	Spoken/Written Instructions	Vague Instructions	Fold socks	15 pairs of socks
3	Confirm understanding	TBD	Feedback (Clear)	Clean table	Cleaner; cloth
4	Confirm understanding	TBD	N/A	Stuff envelopes	15 papers; 15 envelopes
5	Ask for help; Confirm understanding	Spoken/Written Instructions TBD	Vague Instructions	Address envelopes	Address labels; pen

criterion is based on performance across two consecutive opportunities, Bella writes "TBD" for some of the sessions in the "Intervention" column. If Bella's performance does not improve, she will introduce a new intervention.

Step 5: Establish a Plan for Monitoring and Interpreting Performance

Bella will use the template version of the ***Arranged Situations Data Sheet*** to collect data on Michelle's performance during the vague-instructions situation and the ***opportunity-based format*** of the ***Additional Behaviors Data Sheet*** to collect data on confirming statements. Each time Bella gives Michelle an instruction, she will record whether Michelle confirms her understanding.

After each session, Bella will graph Michelle's performance using the percentage-based version of the ***VSSI Graphing Template***. When summarizing the data for the responses involved in asking for help (calling out to Bella within two minutes and emitting an appropriate help statement), Bella will graph 100% if she emits responses both correctly, 50% if she emits just one of the two responses correctly, and 0% if she does not engage in either response. For confirming statements, she will use the "Yes"/"No" feature of this template to indicate whether or not Michelle responded correctly for each opportunity during the appointment.

Step 6: Establish a Plan for Maintenance and Generalization

Next, Bella considers potential strategies for ensuring that Michelle maintains the skills beyond the five scheduled appointments and transfers them to her future new job placements. Before creating a plan, Bella and Michelle use the Identifying Natural Consequences Worksheet in Appendix A to list possible immediate and delayed consequences of engaging in each target or failing to engage in each target. They discuss the possible consequences, shown in Table 12.12. Michelle indicates that she is highly motivated to obtain and maintain a job and that she would like to learn skills that would help her to do so.

However, Bella is concerned about the possible lack of immediate natural reinforcing consequences for confirming understanding of instructions, which she hopes will replace Michelle's inappropriate behavior of complaining or protesting. Thus, if Michelle finds the written instructions beneficial, she will encourage her to review them periodically and to take them with her to future job sites. If Michelle requires BST for any skill, Bella will encourage her to practice the skill(s) periodically with her mother. Finally, regardless of the intervention needed for skill acquisition, Bella also will teach Michelle self-management skills (e.g., goal setting, self-monitoring) to increase the likelihood of both maintenance and generalization.

Table 12.12 Potential naturalistic consequences for Michelle's targeted skills

Target Behavior	What are the immediate and delayed consequences of engaging in the behavior or failing to engage in the behavior?
Confirm understanding	Immediate: No obvious consequences for emitting the target. However, if Michelle does not confirm understanding and complains or protests instead, her supervisor might reprimand or fire her. Delayed: Michelle's relationship with her supervisor might benefit over time if she confirms understanding of instructions.
Ask for help with tasks she doesn't understand	Immediate: Michelle will get the information she needs to complete her work correctly. If she doesn't ask for help, she may have to redo her work. Delayed: Michelle will be considered a valuable employee because she completes her work correctly.

Step 7: Conduct Baseline and Begin Graphing

Bella determines that the data she collected on both targets during the VSSA would be appropriate to use as her baseline for the VSSI. Thus, she begins her graphs by plotting these data. For confirming statements, Bella graphs just the last four opportunities that Michelle had to confirm her understanding of instructions or feedback during the VSSA. Michelle had three opportunities to ask for help during the VSSA, and Bella graphs her performance for each of those opportunities.

Step 8: Conduct the VSSI

Bella begins with the target of asking for help. At the start of the first VSSI appointment, Bell shares her screen to show Michelle the written instructions in Figure 12.16 as she goes over the following spoken instructions for this target:

> *"Sometimes your supervisor may give you a new task without completely describing or showing you how to do it. When this happens, you should ask them to show you how to do it. You can say things like, "Can you should me how?" "I need a model." or "How would you like this done?" Be sure to ask them as soon as possible after you are assigned the task. If you don't ask them to show you how to do the task, you may make mistakes and this may cause problems for the company. You also will need to redo your work. If you ask your supervisor to show you, you will be able to complete the work correctly and your supervisor will think you are a good employee who cares about doing good work.*

If the supervisor gives you a new task without telling or showing you how to do it:

1. Find your supervisor within 2 minutes of the assignment.

2. Ask your supervisor to show you how to do the task. Say

    o Can you show me how"?

    o "I need a model."

    o "How would you like this done?"

Figure 12.16 Written instructions for Michelle during the VSSI.

After ensuring that Michelle understands the instructions and has no more questions, Bella introduces spoken and written instructions for the target of confirming understanding. She uses the same teaching procedures that she did for the first target.

After providing spoken and written instructions for both targets, Bella asks Michelle's mother to print out the written instructions so that Michelle can keep them on the kitchen table while she works. She then tells Michelle that she is going to give her some tasks to complete and that she should practice the skills that they just discussed. Bella reminds Michelle that she will be muting her audio and video feed after giving the instructions for each task but that she can call out if she needs anything. Although Michelle's mother will assist with any technical problems, she will remain in her bedroom during the VSSI appointments.

As Bella conducts the planned VSSI sessions, Michelle's performance on the two skills shows immediate improvement. She meets the acquisition goal for both targets by the end of the second appointment, as shown in the graphs in Figure 12.17. Bella notices that Michelle frequently looks at the written instructions and comments out loud that she is following them. Bella asks Michelle if she likes using the written instructions, and Michelle states that they really help her remember what to do.

Step 9: Assess Maintenance and Generalization

Now that Michelle has met her acquisition goals, Bella continues with the three remaining appointments so that she can assess the short-term maintenance and generalization of the skills. Bella and Michelle discuss the importance of periodically reviewing the written instructions and ways that she might use the written instructions on the job to help her remember to employ the skills. Bella also arranges for one of her colleagues to serve as the supervisor for two work sessions during the fourth appointment so that she can assess Michelle's performance with a new supervisor. Michelle engages in both targets with the colleague, as well.

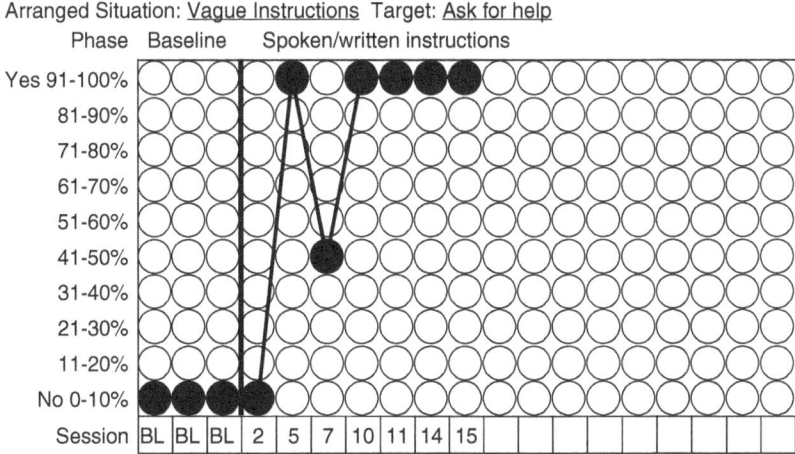

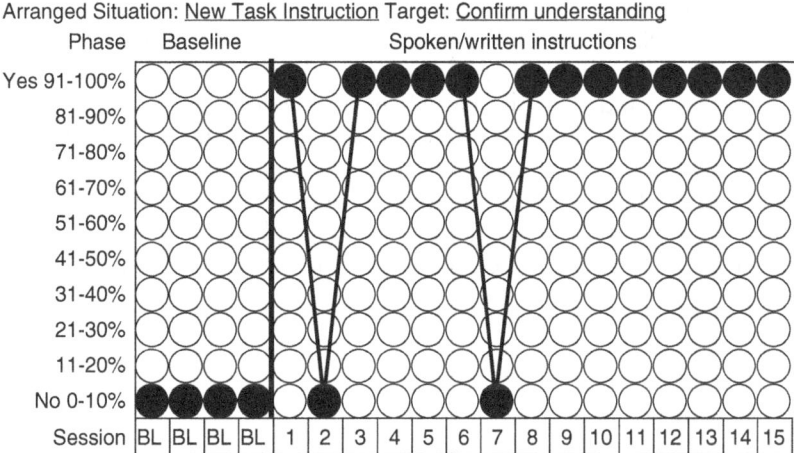

Figure 12.17 Graphs displaying Michelle's performance data for her targeted skills after she receives spoken and written instructions during the VSSI.

In the final appointment with Michelle, Bella discusses the potential benefits of managing her own performance on the job. Michelle indicates an interest in learning how to do so. Given the time constraints, Bella suggests focusing on goal-setting and self-monitoring. As they discuss potential goals for her two targets, Michelle says the maintenance goals from the VSSI were a bit too stringent, as they required correct responses on 100% of opportunities. Instead, Michelle feels as though it would be reasonable if she makes no more than one error per week in asking for help and one error per day in confirming her

When my supervisor gave me a new task without showing me how to do it, I asked her to show me how			Whenever my supervisor gave me an instruction, I let her know that I understood.	
Day	YES	NO	YES	NO

Figure 12.18 Michelle's self-monitoring sheet.

understanding of instructions. Together, they create the self-monitoring sheet shown in Figure 12.18.

Bella uses BST to teach Michelle how to use the self-monitoring sheet and how to determine if she met her goals. First, she models how to use the data sheet, and then she has Michelle practice using it while Bella conducts the remaining planned work sessions. By the end of the appointment, Michelle is monitoring her performance correctly and seems excited about the possibility of using it when she gets a job. Bella reassures Michelle and her mother that she is available to provide further support if Michelle encounters any difficulties after she is placed in her first job.

13 Where to Go from Here? Concluding Comments

The opportunity to participate in meaningful employment can have a tremendous impact on quality of life. In addition to the financial benefits, employment may lead to greater social connections with others and provide the worker with a sense of purpose and accomplishment. Yet, successful employment remains elusive for a substantial number of individuals with NDD who desire the benefits that a job can offer. Numerous families have shared stories about the frustrations, boredom, and loneliness that their adult family member with NDD has experienced due to inadequate preparation for employment. After graduating from high school, many unemployed individuals with NDD remain isolated at home, with few meaningful activities to occupy their time.

Research indicates that a person's social-communication skills are often the linchpin in determining whether they obtain and maintain a job. These skills can be challenging for those with NDD, yet these "soft skills" are frequently overlooked in vocational training programs. In fact, few resources currently exist for professionals who would like to help individuals improve their job-related social and problem-solving skills. It is hoped that this book, with its accompanying protocols and tools, will help to fill this gap.

It is never too soon to start preparing individuals for this important transition to adulthood. A lengthy and diverse set of skills are needed to obtain and maintain employment. Table 13.1 provides just a sample of these myriad, relevant skills. Within the realm of social-communication skills, the first steps should begin in the very early stages of education. Instructors should start by teaching any modality of functional communication that the learner can readily acquire, including vocal or digital speech, picture exchange, or sign language, with an emphasis on teaching the learner to express their wants and needs. At the same time, the instructor should target elementary work skills, such as following instructions, remaining on task for short periods of time, and completing basic occupation-relevant tasks (e.g., sorting, folding, sweeping, cleaning). Once the learner has acquired the minimum prerequisite skills described in Chapter 2, instructors can introduce basic social and problem-solving skills,

DOI: 10.4324/9781003311935-13

Table 13.1 Sample of myriad skills needed to obtain and maintain employment

Answering interview questions	Navigating the job site	Resolving conflicts
Completing applications	Maintaining hygiene	Using safety equipment
Managing time	Selecting appropriate attire	Completing job tasks
Arranging transportation	Requesting time off	Engaging in small talk
Asking for help	Reporting safety concerns	Correcting mistakes

such as greeting others, asking for help when needed, and responding appropriately to feedback.

These basic social and problem-solving skills should be targeted very early in life. Educators and parents can arrange the types of situations described in this book to give the learner opportunities to practice important social-communication skills, such as requesting help with new tasks, confirming understanding of instructions, searching for missing materials, and correcting their mistakes. Table 13.2 lists potential ways to arrange these practice opportunities in the classroom and at home.

When teaching social-communication skills, it is important to individualize the targets and situations to the learner, as illustrated by the case examples in Chapters 7 and 12. The VSSA and VSSI protocols are intended to permit this level of flexibility while still providing a framework that should benefit most learners. For example, targeted communication responses might start with gestures (e.g., pointing to completed work) or simple selection responses (e.g., pointing to a picture of completed work) before progressing to single words or phrases (e.g., saying "Done." or "What next?"), followed by more complex communication (e.g., saying "I finished my work. What should I do next?"). Initial training might prioritize skills that are essential to task completion (e.g., asking for clear instructions, searching for needed materials) before progressing to more complex skills that help build and maintain good social relations (e.g., confirming understanding of instructions, providing unsolicited assistance). At the same time, instructors might start by ensuring that learners encounter basic workplace problems (e.g., finishing a task) before arranging for them to encounter more complex ones (e.g., receiving unclear instructions, running out of materials).

In fact, Table 13.1 suggests that the skills described in this book are just a small portion of those needed to have success in the workplace. The guidelines, procedures, and tools provided with the VSSA and VSSI protocols can be applied when teaching any skill. This includes selecting, defining, and measuring behavior; setting goals; developing and implementing interventions; ensuring maintenance and generalization of skills; and monitoring and evaluating performance.

Finally, close collaboration with the learner is highly recommended when preparing their pathway to employment. Assessing the learner's preferences for different job settings and tasks, along with other aspects of

Table 13.2 Example opportunities for learners to practice job-related social- and problem-solving skills in the classroom and at home

Example Arranged Situation	Potential Targeted Skill(s)
Classroom	
Teacher asks the learner to cut out shapes but does not provide scissors.	Search or ask for needed materials
Teacher interrupts the learner during independent work and asks them to complete a different assignment first.	Switch to new task and return to previous one
Teacher asks the learner to give the class attendance roster to the teaching assistant.	Relay information
Teacher gives the learner a new worksheet to complete without the necessary instructions.	Ask for help
Teacher arranges for a visitor to enter the classroom.	Initiate greetings, wait turn to speak
Teacher tells the learner to take a 5-minute break.	Monitor time
Teachers tells the learner that they completed an assignment incorrectly.	Acknowledge feedback and correct mistakes
Teacher "forgets" to give the learner their assignment for an independent work period.	Ask for next assignment
Teacher spills a box of pencils next to the learner's desk.	Offer assistance
Teacher asks the learner to complete three different tasks during an independent work period.	Transition independently across tasks
Home	
Parent asks the leaner to set the table but does provide enough plates.	Search or ask for needed materials
Parent interrupts the learner while they are completing a chore and asks them to do a different chore first.	Switch to new task and return to previous one
Parent asks the learner to tell another family member that they are going to the store.	Relay information
Parent asks the learner to complete a new chore without providing the necessary instructions.	Ask for help
Parent arranges for a friend to visit the home.	Initiate greetings, wait turn to speak
Parent tells the learner to meet them in the garage in 5 minutes.	Monitor time
Parent tells the learner that they completed a chore incorrectly.	Acknowledge feedback and correct mistakes
Parent helps the learner complete a task.	Thank others
Parent spills a box of envelopes near the learner.	Offer assistance
Parent asks the learner to complete three different chores before leaving the house.	Transition independently across tasks

the work environment, is vital for ensuring that the learner remains motivated to acquire the necessary skills and to perform well once placed on the job (for more information about assessing job preferences see Hall et al., 2014; Ninci et al., 2017; St. Peter et al., 2022; Tullis & Seaman-Tullis, 2019; Walsh et al., 2020). The learner's input and preferences should be incorporated into the selected goals, situations, and interventions whenever possible. By working together, the learner and those who strive to see them succeed can make their long-term employment goals and dreams a reality.

Reference List

Hall, J., Morgan, R. L., & Salzberg, C. L. (2014). Job-preference and job-matching assessment results and their association with job performance and satisfaction among young adults with developmental disabilities. *Education and Training in Autism and Developmental Disabilities*, 301–312.

Ninci, J., Gerow, S., Rispoli, M., & Boles, M. (2017). Systematic review of vocational preferences on behavioral outcomes of individuals with disabilities. *Journal of Developmental and Physical Disabilities*, *29*(6), 875–894.

St Peter, C., Shuler, N. J., Toegel, C., Diaz-Salvat, C., & Jones, S. H. (2022). Using preference assessments to identify preferred job tasks for adolescents with autism. *Education and Treatment of Children*, *45*(1), 17–32.

Tullis, C. A., & Seaman-Tullis, R. L. (2019). Incorporating preference assessment into transition planning for people with autism spectrum disorder. *Behavior Analysis in Practice*, *12*(3), 727–733.

Walsh, E., Lydon, H., & Holloway, J. (2020). An evaluation of assistive technology in determining job-specific preference for adults with autism and intellectual disabilities. *Behavior Analysis in Practice*, *13*(2), 434–444.

Appendix A

1. Reinforcer Survey
2. Preference Assessment Instructions and Data Sheets
3. Pre-Assessment Interview Form
4. Employer Interview Form
5. Other Situations Quick Reference Tables
6. Potential Tasks and Materials List
7. VSSA Plan Template
8. Defining Behaviors
9. Identifying Naturalistic Consequences Worksheet

1. Reinforcer Survey

REINFORCER SURVEY					
Name: _____ Date: _____ Completed by:					

Instructions: Professionals should interview the learner to identify potential reinforcers that may be utilized when teaching new skills. In the section below, determine which general categories are of most interest. Many choices below are not immediately available at most worksites, but may serve as delayed, larger reinforcers for learners at work or home. Speak to caregivers about the possibility of including non-worksite reinforcers into the learner's program.

1: *"I don't like it at all."*		2: *"I only sometimes like it."*		3: *"I love it."*	

Activity, Food, or Item					
SNACKS AND BEVERAGES			**HOBBIES AND LEISURE ACTIVITIES**		
Soft Drinks (Soda)	1 2 3		Take walks	1 2 3	
Lemonade or Tea	1 2 3		Play cards or board games	1 2 3	
Sparking or flavored waters	1 2 3		Create art/drawing/jewelry/crafts	1 2 3	
Milk or Chocolate Milk	1 2 3		Rest and closing eyes	1 2 3	
Salty Snacks	1 2 3		Read books or magazines	1 2 3	
Fast Foods	1 2 3		Assemble a puzzle	1 2 3	
Fruits or Vegetables	1 2 3		**DELAYED, LARGER REINFORCERS**		
Desserts	1 2 3		Visit a restaurant	1 2 3	
Nuts	1 2 3		Ride a bike	1 2 3	
TECHNOLOGY			Shop	1 2 3	
Listen to music	1 2 3		Go to the movies	1 2 3	
Take pictures	1 2 3		Attend a sports game	1 2 3	
Watch TV/movies on a tablet	1 2 3		**SOCIAL CONNECTIONS**		
Watch how-to videos	1 2 3		Call a family member or friend	1 2 3	
Play online games	1 2 3		Receive a compliment	1 2 3	
Type on a keyboard	1 2 3		Do errands or be helpful	1 2 3	
Reading about favorite topics	1 2 3		Receive a High 5	1 2 3	
Edit photos	1 2 3		Talk to friends	1 2 3	
Text with friends or family	1 2 3		Visit a favorite adult	1 2 3	
JOB-RELATED REWARDS					
Positive performance evaluation	1 2 3		"Late Arrival to Work" pass	1 2 3	
Longer breaks from work	1 2 3		"Early Dismissal from Work" pass	1 2 3	
More frequent breaks from work	1 2 3		Extra vacation days	1 2 3	
Choice of work tasks	1 2 3		Earn money/gift cards to shop at stores	1 2 3	
"Skip a Task" Card	1 2 3		Earn tokens or tickets for rewards	1 2 3	

Notes:

2. Preference Assessment Instructions and Data Sheets

How to Conduct A Preference Assessment: The Multiple-Stimulus-Without-Replacement (MSWO)[1] Format

The following is a brief overview of recommended steps and tips for conducting a preference assessment called the Multiple Stimulus Without Replacement (MSWO) Assessment and a data sheet for recording and interpreting the outcomes

HOW TO CONDUCT A PREFERENCE ASSESSMENT
Preparing for the Assessment
Identify up to 7 potential reinforcers for the learner by having them or those who know them complete a reinforcer survey
Identify a space at a table that is free of visual and audible distractions
Collect up to 7 potential reinforcing items or use pictures of activities that cannot be brought to the table
If assessing food, cut or portion into small, equal servings.
List the name of each item, food, or activity in a separate box across the data sheet
Assessing Preferred Items, Food, or Activities as Potential Reinforcers
Arrange the items or pictures approximately 2" apart in a line on the table in front of the learner
Say, "pick one!" and permit the learner to select from the array
Allow 30 seconds-2 minutes with the item/activity, or bite of food; note choice on data sheet (Trial 1)
Ask learner to return item and remove the item/picture from future rotation
Initiate Trial 2 by rearranging remaining items/pictures in a line and permit learner to choose one again
Continue recording selections and presenting remaining items/pictures until no items are left or the learner does not choose any of the remaining items/pictures
Repeat assessment several times, each one at least 24 hours apart.
Determining Preferences
Typically, items chosen in earlier trials are most preferred, whereas items chosen in the later trials are least preferred. Make a note of the items, food, or activities that the learner usually selects in the first 3 trials. It is important to reassess preferences regularly.
Troubleshooting and Tips for Success
If the learner approaches two items simultaneously, prevent the learner from accessing either item and ask the learner to choose just one
Keep items and portions similar size. Assess food preferences separately from item and activity preferences.
Randomize the order of items during each trial.
Conduct a full assessment (offering each item) 3-5 times for most accurate results
If the learner fails to select an item or food, instruct again to "pick one." If no choice is made after 5-10 seconds, note "no choice" on the remainder of the options and terminate the assessment.
Refrain from praising particular selections or encouraging some items over others to avoid biasing the results

---

[1] For additional information, consult DeLeon, I. G., & Iwata, B. A. (1996). Evaluation of a multiple-stimulus presentation format for assessing reinforcer preferences. *Journal of applied behavior analysis, 29*(4), 519-533.

MULTIPLE STIMULUS WITHOUTREPLACEMENT (MSWO) PREFERENCE ASSESSMENT DATA SHEET							
Name: _____ Date: _____ Completed by: _____							
Instructions: Place an "X" under the item chosen on each trial. For each trial, omit all previously selected items.							
ITEMS							
List up to 7 items across the top							
Trial 1							
Trial 2							
Trial 3							
Trial 4							
Trial 5							
Trial 6							
Trial 7							
List items consistently selected first, second, and third:							
Notes:							

3. Pre-Assessment Interview Form

PRE-ASSESSMENT INTERVIEW	
Instructions: This form may be helpful when gathering information about the learner. The information collected may help guide vocational assessments, job placements, and intervention plans. Schedule a meeting with the learner and others who are familiar with them . Read or paraphrase the questions and record responses on this form. **Throughout this form, "you" refers to the learner.**	
Your name:	Caregiver's name (if applicable):
Your phone number:	Your birthday:
Your email:	Any Diagnoses:
Your home address:	
List medications and all treatments you receive:	
Hobbies and Interests	
What hobbies do you enjoy?	
Do you enjoy time with friends?	
Vocational Interests and Employment Preparedness	
Where would you like to work?	
Where do you NOT want to work? Why?	
Would you prefer to work alone or with others?	
How do you receive money to spend?	
Do you receive Social Security benefits?	
Home LIfe	
What do you spend your money on?	
How do you get to places you want to go (does someone drive you)?	
How do you wake up in the morning (e.g. alarm clock, someone wakes you)?	
What does your typical day look like?	
Morning:	Afternoon:	Evening:
How do you keep yourself organized (e.g., planner, calendar)?	
What chores or responsibilities are assigned to you at home ?	
Where will you live in the future?	
Education	
What is your highest level of education completed (e.g., high school diploma)?	
What, if any, supports did you receive in school?	
What are your post-graduation goals?	

Work and Volunteer History
Describe the job training that you received in the past.
Describe any interviews that you have done.
Have you ever done a mock interview for practice?
Describe your prior work/volunteer experience.
List all past employment (jobs).

Hours per week?		Duration of job:	Responsibilities:		Why did you leave your job?

What are you good at in your job?
What is hardest for you at work?

Do you have experience with the following ?

Staple papers	Sort mail	Fold papers	Make boxes	Use a cash register
Stack items	Put files away	Stuff envelopes	Fold clothes	Count money
Sort papers	Hang clothes	Sort silverware	Put prices on items	Prepare food

What other experience do you have?

Job-related Social Skills
How are your interactions with coworkers ?
How are your interactions with your supervisors?
Do you interact with customers? If so, how are those interactions?
How do you typically handle corrective feedback?
What do you do if someone (e.g., parents) ask s you to do something that you do not want to do?
What do you do when you do not know how to do something?

Computer
If you have an email address, how often do you use it?
Describe any experience you have with computer software, such as Microsoft Word, Excel, and PowerPoint. .
Can you use search engines (e.g., Google) to research things?

Telling Time
Can you read a digital or analog clock to tell time?
Can you tell what time it will be in 10 minutes?

The questions in the following two sections should be directed to caregivers or other adults who are familiar with the learner:

Reading, Writing, and Communication Skills
Describe the learner's reading level.
Describe the learner's writing skills.
How does the learner communicate their wants and needs (e.g., complete sentences, short statements, picture communication, etc)/How are their conversation skills?

Potentially Challenging Behaviors
What, if any, behavior challenges has your learner experienced while at home or in the community (ex: difficulty remaining on task, making inappropriate comments, crying, leaving the area)
Does the learner engage in inappropriate behavior when no one is around, with everyone around, or only in the presence of certain people?
Does the learner engage in inappropriate behavior if an activity, food, or item is unavailable or denied (ex: the learner is told no or to wait)?
Does the learner engage in inappropriate behavior if a preferred activity is interrupted or removed?
Does the learner engage in inappropriate behavior when asked to complete a task or do something that is nonpreferred (ex: hygiene or other routines, routines, chores, attend medical appointments)?
Does the learner engage in inappropriate behavior following attempts to gain attention, or after a period of time when no attention has been given?
When the learner engages in inappropriate behavior, do people in the environment provide attention, either verbally or physically?
When the learner engages in inappropriate behavior, do people in the environment attempt to soothe the learner by providing preferred items, or redirect them to food and activities?
When the learner engages in inappropriate behavior, do people in the environment give the learner a break or remove chores, expectations of work, or a nonpreferred situation?
Does the learner appear to experience sensitivity to noises, lights, smells, or other environmental stressors?
What supports or interventions have been tried? Discuss the learner's experience with the interventions.

4. Employer Interview Form

Employer Survey/Interview Form

Interviewee Name/Title:

Name of Company:

Targeted Position Title and Responsibilities:

We are interested in getting more information about the position and work environment at your company and the social- and problem-solving skills that employees in this position need to be successful at your organization.

1 Have you ever worked with an employee with a neurodevelopmental disability, such as autism spectrum disorder or intellectual disabilities? If so, can you briefly describe your experience?

2 Will the employee have to interact with customers? If so, please describe the nature of these interactions.

3 Will the employee have to work with others to complete their responsibilities? If so, please describe the nature of this teamwork.

4 Describe the pace of the work (e.g., fast, moderate, slow) and time constraints.

5 Describe the predictability of the schedule and work routine (e.g., very predictable, somewhat predictable, very unpredictable).

6 Describe other aspects of the work environment in terms of lighting (e.g., dim, bright, harsh, soft) and sounds (e.g., quiet, loud).

7 Please rate the importance of each of the following social- and problem-solving skills for the employee who will be filling this position. Using the following rating scale, select your rating by placing an "X" in the appropriate box at the end of each description:
        1 = not at all important
        2 = slightly important
        3 = somewhat important
        4 = very important
        5 = extremely important

Rate the importance of the following skills in your place of business:	1	2	3	4	5
The employee confirms understanding when they are given a new task (e.g., "Got it!" "Ok! I will do that!").					
The employee asks for clarification when they do not understand how to do a task.					
The employee independently obtains materials that they need to complete a task without having to get assistance from others.					
The employee asks for help if missing or broken materials prevent them from completing a task.					
The employee lets the supervisor know when they have completed a task.					
The employee asks the supervisor what they should do next when they have finished their assigned tasks.					
The employee finds other work to do when supervisors or co-workers are unavailable to help them solve a problem with their current task.					
The employee immediately switches to a newly assigned task when asked to do so.					
The employee acknowledges corrective feedback (e.g., "Thank you for letting me know!" "Sorry for the error!") when they are told to do the work differently.					
The employee confirms that they will correct their mistakes ("Got it!" "I will do that!") when they are given corrective feedback.					
The employee compliments co-workers.					
The employee offers to help other co-workers when needed.					
The employee knocks on closed office doors and waits for a response before entering.					
The employee returns from breaks on time.					
The employee works at a faster pace when told that the work needs to be completed more quickly or when given a deadline that must be met.					
The employee reports problems that they observe on the job (e.g., damaged or malfunctioning equipment, spills).					
The employee waits for others to stop speaking before making a comment or question (i.e., the employee does not interrupt others).					
The employee says "please" and "thank you" when appropriate.					
The employee says "excuse me" or apologizes when appropriate (e.g., when interrupting someone's work, when accidentally bumping into someone).					
The employee remains focused and calm despite personal issues or stressors.					
The employee remains calm and focused despite disruptions on the job (e.g., changes in routine, interruptions by co-workers.					
The employee accurately relays information to others.					
The employee engages in appropriate small talk with co-workers.					
The employee engages in appropriate small talk with customers.					
The employee makes eye contact when speaking with others.					

8 What do you think are the most important social and problem-solving skills for the employee in this position?

9 What are the biggest barriers to your employees' success on the job?

10 What are the most common reasons that employees in this position are not successful?

11 Is there anything else that you think we should know about the position and how best to support potential employees?

5. Other Situations Quick Reference Tables

Example quick reference tables for additional situations that instructors could include in the VSSA

Instructed to Relay Information		
Supervisor: Instruct the learner to seek out and relay information to another person. The response can involve relaying information vocally, via written materials, or both, depending on the skills of the learner. Terminate situation by instructing learner to resume previous task or to complete a new task if they remain off task for more than 5 minutes.		
Learner Behavior	**Definition**	**Opportunities to Collect Data**
1. Seeks person	Learner starts to search for the person within 1 minute of receiving the instruction	Any time the learner is told to relay information to someone
2. Relays information correctly	Learner accurately conveys the information in the manner requested	Any time the learner locates the targeted recipient of information.
3. Returns to work	Learner resumes assigned work or asks the supervisor what they should do next within 1 minute of relaying information or failing to locate the recipient.	Any time the learner relays information to recipient or fails to locate the recipient.

Assigned Multiple Tasks (Fixed or Unfixed Sequence)		
Supervisor: Select at least two tasks that the learner should complete. Give the learner clear instructions about the tasks and indicate desired order of completion (if fixed sequence). End the situation when the learner has completed all of the tasks, indicates that they are finished, or remains idle for more than 2 minutes. Optional: Provide a written list of the tasks		
Learner Behavior	**Definition**	**Opportunities to Collect Data**
Transitions to Next Task	Learner starts next assigned task within 2 minutes of completing the previous one. NOTE: If using a fixed sequence, only score as correct if task is completed in desired order.	Any time the learner completes a task, regardless of whether the task was completed correctly.

Supervisor/Co-Worker Needs Assistance (Unsolicited)		
Supervisor/Co-Worker: Demonstrate a clear need for assistance within eyesight of the learner without verbally requesting assistance. For example, attempt to lift a heavy box, spill items, etc. Terminate after 1 minute if the learner does not offer assistance.		
Learner Behavior	**Definition**	**Opportunities to Collect Data**
1. Offers Assistance	Asks the person if they can help.	Any time someone demonstrates need for assistance
2. Provides Assistance	Provides assistance for an appropriate amount of time.	Any time the learner offers assistance and the person accepts
3. Responds to Gratitude	Says "you are welcome," or any other relevant, appropriate statement.	Any time the person makes a gratitude statement following assistance
4. Returns to Work	Returns to previous work task after providing assistance	Any time learner provides assistance

Supervisor/Co-Worker Needs Assistance (Solicited)		
Supervisor/Co-Worker: Ask the learner for brief assistance with a task (e.g., help pick up spilled items)		
Learner Behavior	Definition	Opportunities to Collect Data
1. Acknowledges Request	Provides relevant affirmation statement	Any time someone requests assistance
2. Provides Assistance	Provides assistance for an appropriate amount of time	Any time someone requests assistance
3. Responds to Gratitude	Says "you are welcome," or any other relevant, appropriate statement.	Any time the person makes a gratitude statement following assistance
4. Returns to Work	Returns to previous work task after providing assistance	Any time learner provides assistance

Provided Compliment		
Supervisor / Co-Worker: Deliver a statement of admiration in reference to the learner's behavior (e.g., completing high-quality work) or an item in the person's possession (e.g., article of clothing, accessory)		
Learner Behavior	Definition	Opportunities to Collect Data
Expresse s gratitude	Says "thank you" or other relevant, appropriate statement	Any time the learner is given a compliment

End of Break		
Supervisor: Inform the learner that they may take a break of a certain length. Instruct the learner to either return to work or to find the supervisor for the next assignment at the end of the break. End the break by asking the learner to return to work if they have not resumed work within 5 minutes of the end of the break.		
Learner Behavior	Definition	Opportunities to Collect Data
Resumes Work	Learner returns to their assigned tasks or requests their next assignment within 2 minutes of the end of the designated break time	Any time the learner is told to task a certain length break.

6. Potential Tasks and Materials List

Potential Tasks and Materials List

The following is a list of possible tasks grouped by industry area with associated materials, suggested instructions when arranging the vague-instructions or task-not-in-repertoire situations, and recommended ways to arrange the materials-needed situation for that task. Tasks that require tools (e.g., hammer, saw, drill) should only be assigned with adequate protective equipment and to learners with demonstrated ability to use the tools safely,

Clerical/Office Tasks:

Scheduling
Materials: Computer or laptop with a calendar and document(s) with dates/times of appointments, daily menus, etc.
For Vague Instructions / Task Not In Repertoire Situation: Say "Make a calendar" or "complete this scheduling" without providing additional instructions or a model. For Materials Needed Situation: Omit calendar or needed documents

Filing
Materials: File box or drawer, stack of documents that could be filed by name, date, color, content, etc.
For Vague Instructions / Task Not In Repertoire Situation: Say "File" without indicating whether to file by name, date, color, content, etc. For Materials Needed Situation: Omit the file box, folders, or dividers

Faxing
Materials: Fax machine, fax number(s), document(s)
For Vague Instructions / Task Not In Repertoire Situation: Say "Fax" without providing additional instructions or a model. For Materials Needed Situation: Omit fax number(s); disable fax machine

Laminating
Materials: Laminating machine, paper(s) to laminate; lamination covers
For Vague Instructions / Task Not In Repertoire Situation: Say "Laminate" without providing additional instructions or a model. For Materials Needed Situation: Omit the lamination covers; disable the laminator

Organizing Binders/Files
Materials: Set of binders/files that could be organized by name, date, color, content, etc.; shelf/box to place them
For Vague Instructions / Task Not In Repertoire Situation: Say "Organize these binders (or files)" without indicating whether to organize by name, data, color, content, etc. For Materials Needed Situation: Include some damaged files or binders

Stapling or Paper Clipping Documents
Materials: Two or more stacks of documents. Stapler or box of paper clips.
For Vague Instructions / Task Not In Repertoire Situation: Say "Staple these documents" or "paper clip these documents" without indicating the order or number of documents to collate; where to place the staple or paper clip, etc. For Materials Needed Situation: Provide an inadequate number of staples or paperclips; include some damaged documents; provide an unequal number of documents.

Proofreading Documents
Materials: Electronic or hard-copy document with grammar and spelling errors
For Vague Instructions / Task Not In Repertoire Situation: Say "proofread" or "find the errors" without providing additional instructions or a model. Materials Needed Situation: Omit pen/pencil or dictionary

Editing Documents
Materials: Electronic document; list of necessary edits (e.g., change font size or style; center and underline all headings, re-organize sections, etc).
For Vague Instructions / Task Not In Repertoire Situation: Say "make these changes" without providing additional instructions or a model. Materials Needed Situation: N/A

Removing Staples
Materials: Stapled papers, stapler remover
For Vague Instructions / Task Not In Repertoire Situation: Say "Remove the staples" without providing additional instructions or a model For Materials Needed Situation: Omit staple remover

Scanning Documents
Materials: Scanner, papers to scan
For Vague Instructions / Task Not In Repertoire Situation: Say "scan" without providing additional instructions or a model. For Materials Needed Situation: Disable scanner

Printing Documents
Materials: Files to print; printer
For Vague Instructions / Task Not In Repertoire Situation: Say "print these documents" without providing additional instructions or a model. For Materials Needed Situation: Disable printer; provide inadequate amount of paper

Stuffing Envelopes
Materials: Documents, envelopes
For Vague Instructions / Task Not In Repertoire Situation: Say "Stuff the envelopes" without additional instruction or a model For Materials Needed Situation: Don't provide enough envelopes; include damaged envelops or documents

Transcribing
Materials: Computer and document(s)
For Vague Instructions / Task Not In Repertoire Situation: Say "transcribe this" without additional instruction or a model For Materials Needed Situation: Hide or remove word-processing application/software from computer

Addressing Envelopes
Materials: List of addresses, pen, address labels, envelopes
For Vague Instructions / Task Not In Repertoire Situation: Say "address the envelopes" without additional instruction or a model For Materials Needed Situation: Omit addresses, pen, labels, or envelopes; provide inadequate number of labels

Shredding
Materials: Stack of documents to shred; shredder
For Vague Instructions / Task Not In Repertoire Situation: Say "shred" without providing additional instructions or a model. For Materials Needed Situation: Disable the shredder

Creating Binders
Materials: Three-ring binders, dividers, documents
For Vague Instructions / Task Not In Repertoire Situation: Say "put together these binders" without providing additional instructions or a model. For Materials Needed Situation: Provide an inadequate number of dividers or documents

Entering Data
<u>Materials</u>: Computer; spreadsheet; hard copy document with data (e.g., mileage, hours worked, inventory, etc)
<u>For Vague Instructions / Task Not In Repertoire Situation</u>: Say "enter these data" without providing additional instructions or a model. <u>For Materials Needed Situation</u>: Hide or remove spreadsheet; omit some necessary data

Calculating Data
<u>Materials</u>: Computer; spreadsheet with information on mileage, payroll or other computational data
<u>For Vague Instructions / Task Not In Repertoire Situation</u>: Say "calculate <name>" without providing additional instructions or a model. <u>For Materials Needed Situation</u>: Omit some necessary data

Graphing Data
<u>Materials</u>: Computer or graph paper; graphing software; data sets
<u>For Vague Instructions / Task Not In Repertoire Situation</u>: Say "graph these data" without providing additional instructions or a model. <u>For Materials Needed Situation</u>: Omit graph paper (for hard copy graphs); hide or remove graphing software from computer; omit some necessary data

Researching
<u>Materials</u>: Computer with internet access; wording processing software; topic to research (e.g.., top ten highest paying jobs, population numbers.)
<u>For Vague Instructions / Task Not In Repertoire Situation</u>: Say "Find information on <topic>" without providing additional instructions or a model. <u>For Materials Needed Situation</u>: Disable internet access

Retail:

Alphabetizing/Organizing Books
Materials: Books and shelves, bin, or cart
For Vague Instructions / Task Not In Repertoire Situation: Say "organize" or "alphabetize these books" without saying whether to arrange by author name, title, etc For Materials Needed Situation: N/A
Bagging Supplies or Purchases
Materials: Office supplies (pens, pencils, highlighters, notepads), Ziploc bags/pencil pouches, grocery items, tote bags/plastic grocery bags
For Vague Instructions / Task Not In Repertoire Situation: Say "make supply bags" without indicating what to put in each bag or "bag these items" without further instruction. For Materials Needed Situation: Provide inadequate number of bags or unequal number of items (for supply bags); provide broken or damaged bags or items
Making Invoices
Materials: Computer with invoice template; document(s) with information on items purchased
For Vague Instructions / Task Not In Repertoire Situation: Say "create invoices" without further instruction or a model. For Materials Needed Situation: Omit template; omit information on items purchased
Hanging or Folding Clothing
Materials: Clothing (shirts, shorts, pants, etc), hangers, clothes rack
For Vague Instructions / Task Not In Repertoire Situation: Say "fold these" or "hang these up" without further instruction or a model. For Materials Needed Situation: Provide insufficient number of hangers, include broken hangers
Matching/Folding Socks
Materials: Various different pairs of socks (colors, styles, etc)
For Vague Instructions / Task Not In Repertoire Situation: Say "match these" or "fold these" without further instruction or a model. For Materials Needed Situation: Omit some matching socks
Pricing Items
Materials: Pricing stickers (with or without price pre-printed), supplies, groceries items
For Vague Instructions / Task Not In Repertoire Situation: Say "price these" without additional instructions about pricing of items or desired location of stickers. For Materials Needed Situation: Omit some prices (pre-printed stickers), provide inadequate number of stickers
Stocking
Materials: Various grocery or retail items, shelving unit or storage cabinet with drawers
For Vague Instructions / Task Not In Repertoire Situation: Say "stock" or "put these away" without instructions on where to place items or how to arrange them. For Materials Needed Situation: N/A
Taking Inventory
Materials: Various grocery or retail items (on table, in boxes, on shelves, in drawers); inventory sheet, pen, clipboard
For Vague Instructions / Task Not In Repertoire Situation: Say "take inventory" without further instructions or modeling. For Materials Needed Situation: Omit inventory sheet or pen

Janitorial:

Dusting
<u>Materials</u>: Dust cloth, dusty areas/objects
<u>For Vague Instructions / Task Not In Repertoire Situation</u>: Say "dust" without further instructions or modeling on what to do or what to dust.   <u>For Materials Needed Situation</u>: Omit cloth

Sweeping / Vacuuming
<u>Materials</u>: Broom and dustpan; vacuum
<u>For Vague Instructions / Task Not In Repertoire Situation</u>: Say "sweep" or vacuum without further instructions or modeling.   <u>For Materials Needed Situation</u>: Omit broom, dustpan, or vacuum

Mopping
<u>Materials</u>: Mop, bucket, soap
<u>For Vague Instructions / Task Not In Repertoire Situation</u>: Say "mop" without further instructions or modeling.   <u>For Materials Needed Situation</u>: Omit mop, bucket, or soap

Sanitizing Surfaces
<u>Materials</u>: cleaning wipes, spray or other cleaner, towels
<u>For Vague Instructions / Task Not In Repertoire Situation</u>: Say "clean" without further instructions or modeling on what to do or what to clean.   <u>For Materials Needed Situation</u>: Omit wipes, cleaner, etc.

Doing Laundry
<u>Materials</u>: Cloth items to be washed (towels, sheets, clothing); laundry basket; washer and dryer; soap; dryer sheets
<u>For Vague Instructions / Task Not In Repertoire Situation</u>: Say "do this laundry" without further instruction or modeling   <u>For Materials Needed Situation</u>: Omit soap or dryer sheets; unplug washer or dryer

Warehouse/Backroom:

Assembling Boxes
<u>Materials</u>: Boxes, tape (if needed)
<u>For Vague Instructions / Task Not In Repertoire Situation</u>: Say "make these boxes" without further instruction or modeling   <u>For Materials Needed Situation</u>: Omit tape (if needed); include damaged boxes

Labeling
<u>Materials</u>: Label maker or labels and pen; boxes/bins with assorted items
<u>For Vague Instructions / Task Not In Repertoire Situation</u>: Say "label these boxes" without further instruction or modeling   <u>For Materials Needed Situation</u>: Omit labels, label maker, or pen

Packing
<u>Materials</u>: Packing material (Styrofoam, bubble wrap), boxes; tape; assorted items to pack
<u>For Vague Instructions / Task Not In Repertoire Situation</u>: Say "pack these" without further instruction or modeling   <u>For Materials Needed Situation</u>: Omit tape, provide inadequate amount of packing material or boxes; include damaged boxes

Stacking/Moving Boxes
<u>Materials</u>: Labeled boxes, shelving units
<u>For Vague Instructions / Task Not In Repertoire Situation</u>: Say "stack" or "move" the boxes without further instruction or modeling   <u>For Materials Needed Situation</u>: N/A

Food Industry

Busing Tables
Materials: Tables with dishes; container; cloth; cleaner
For Vague Instructions / Task Not In Repertoire Situation: Say "bus these tables" without further instruction or modeling For Materials Needed Situation: Omit dish container, cloth, cleaner

Taking Orders
Materials: Order pad, pen
For Vague Instructions / Task Not In Repertoire Situation: Say "take these (pretend) customer orders" without further instruction or modeling For Materials Needed Situation: Omit pad or pen

Prepping Food
Materials: Knife set; cutting board; food safety gloves; storage containers with lids; various fruits, vegetables or cheeses
For Vague Instructions / Task Not In Repertoire Situation: Say "prep these" without further instruction or modeling For Materials Needed Situation: Omit knives, cutting board, or containers

Putting Dishes Away
Materials: Various plates, cups, cutlery; storage cabinet or shelves
For Vague Instructions / Task Not In Repertoire Situation: Say "put these away" without further instruction on where to place items or how to arrange them For Materials Needed Situation: N/A

Making Simple Sandwiches
Materials: A list of sandwiches to prepare; necessary food(s) to prepare the sandwiches; saran wrap/to-go boxes, food safety gloves
For Vague Instructions / Task Not In Repertoire Situation: Say "makes these sandwiches" without further instruction or modeling For Materials Needed Situation: Omit list of sandwiches to prepare; omit bread or other necessary ingredient; provide inadequate amount of ingredients or to-go boxes

Restocking Table Caddy/Condiment Holder
Materials: Condiment bottles; various condiments
For Vague Instructions / Task Not In Repertoire Situation: Say "refill these bottles" without further instruction or modeling For Materials Needed Situation: Provide inadequate amounts of condiments

Rolling Silverware
Materials: Cloth or paper napkins; silverware (forks, knives, spoons)
For Vague Instructions / Task Not In Repertoire Situation: Say "roll the silverware" without further instruction or modeling For Materials Needed Situation: Provide inadequate number of napkins; include some torn or damaged napkins; provide unequal number of forks, knives, and spoons

Setting Table(s)
Materials: Plates, cups, silverware, table(s) with chairs.
For Vague Instructions / Task Not In Repertoire Situation: Say "set the tables" without further instruction or modeling For Materials Needed Situation: Provide inadequate number of dishes or silverware.

Washing Dishes
Materials: Various dishes, pots, silverware; dish soap; sponge; dish drainer
For Vague Instructions / Task Not In Repertoire Situation: Say "wash the dishes" without further instruction or modeling For Materials Needed Situation: Omit soap, sponge, or dish drainer

Construction/Maintenance:

Assembling Furniture
<u>Materials</u>: Furniture kits, written instructions, necessary tools
<u>For Vague Instructions / Task Not In Repertoire Situation</u>: Say "assemble the \<furniture name\> without further instruction or modeling <u>For Materials Needed Situation</u>: Omit written instructions, necessary tool

Drilling Holes
<u>Materials</u>: Drill, wooden board with marked hole placements
<u>For Vague Instructions / Task Not In Repertoire Situation</u>: Say "drill the holes" without further instruction or modeling <u>For Materials Needed Situation</u>: Omit drill or wooden board

Hammering Nails
<u>Materials</u>: Hammer, nails, wooden board with marked nail placements
<u>For Vague Instructions / Task Not In Repertoire Situation</u>: Say "hammer the nails" without further instruction or modeling <u>For Materials Needed Situation</u>: Omit hammer, provide inadequate number of nails

Inserting Screws
<u>Materials</u>: Screws, screwdriver, board with pre-drilled holes
<u>For Vague Instructions / Task Not In Repertoire Situation</u>: Say "insert the screws" without further instruction or modeling <u>For Materials Needed Situation</u>: Omit screwdriver or provide the wrong type of screwdriver, provide inadequate number of screws

Securing Nuts and Bolts
<u>Materials</u>: Set of bolts with fasteners
<u>For Vague Instructions / Task Not In Repertoire Situation</u>: Say "put together the nuts and bolts" without further instruction or modeling <u>For Materials Needed Situation</u>: Provide inadequate number of fasteners

Testing Batteries
<u>Materials</u>: Batteries, battery tester
<u>For Vague Instructions / Task Not In Repertoire Situation</u>: Say "test the batters" without further instruction or modeling <u>For Materials Needed Situation</u>: Omit the battery tester

Taping
<u>Materials</u>: Tape (electrical, insulation, masking, or duct); plastic tubes or pipes; piece or wood to be painted
<u>For Vague Instructions / Task Not In Repertoire Situation</u>: Say "tape this" without further instruction or modeling <u>For Materials Needed Situation</u>: Provide an inadequate amount of tape.

Painting
<u>Materials</u>: Paint, brushes, roller, wood or other objects to paint
<u>For Vague Instructions / Task Not In Repertoire Situation</u>: Say "paint this" without further instruction or modeling <u>For Materials Needed Situation</u>: Omit brush; provide inadequate amount of paint

Sawing
<u>Materials</u>: Saw, wood with markings, sawhorse or table
<u>For Vague Instructions / Task Not In Repertoire Situation</u>: Say "saw this" without further instruction or modeling <u>For Materials Needed Situation</u>: Omit saw

7. VSSA Plan Template

VSSA Plan

Learner: _____ Instructor: _____

Assessment Dates: _____

Session #	Task(s)	Arranged Situation(s)	Materials Needed

8. Defining Behaviors

GUIDELINES FOR DEFINING BEHAVIOR
Creating operational definitions of behaviors is important for determining exactly what you plan to target and for collecting reliable, accurate data on performance. Definitions should have the following characteristics: Objective – Definitions should include only physical characteristics of the behavior that can be observed and measured. Clear – Definitions should be unambiguous so that everyone reading the definition understands what is being targeted for change and will collect data in the same way Complete - Definitions should include both examples of the target behavior as well as relevant examples that should be excluded from the definition.

EXAMPLES OF MEASUREABLE, OBSERVABLE TARGET BEHAVIORS		
Lays head on table	Swipes items from table	Slams hand on surfaces
Walks away from work area	Talks on the phone	Says "thank you."
Uses swear words	Engages in name-calling	Offers to help

EXAMPLES OF SUBJECTIVE, NON-OBSERVABLE BEHAVIORS*		
Frustrated	Tired and upset	Lazy
Angry	Acting silly	Sad
Feelings are hurt	Seeking revenge	Anxious

*These descriptors do not aid in adequately establishing a concrete and objective data collection system.

EXAMPLES OF EXCLUSIONS FROM DEFINITION BASED UPON CONTEXT	
Yelling does not count while outside or during recreation	Leaving area does not count when on breaks, seeking supervisor, or end of shift
Open-hand strikes do not count when giving Hi-5s	Responding with "no" is only counted when a work task has been presented; other contexts should not be considered "refusals"
Crying does not count when injured	Destroying papers does not count when the paper belongs to the learner

TEMPLATE FOR WRITING DEFINITIONS AND EXAMPLES
(Name of Behavior) occurs when the learner *(insert the objective description of the behavior with actions that can be observed and counted or measured)*, *(under a certain context, if applicable)*. The behavior should not be counted as occurring if *(list exceptions)*.

9. Identifying Naturalistic Consequences Worksheet

IDENTIFING NATURAL CONSEQUENCES WORKSHEET

Learner's Name: Person Completing Form: Date:

It is important to identify potential reinforcing consequences that might maintain performance in the job setting beyond any support arranged by the instructor. To better determine whether the learner's behavior is likely to receive effective, naturalistic reinforcement on the job, address the questions in this worksheet for each targeted skill. If it isn't clear that a behavior will result in reinforcing consequences for the learner, try to ensure that the learner receives some type of reward for their efforts. See Chapters 3 and 11.

Target Behavior	What typically happens when workers engage in this behavior or fail to engage in this behavior? How do supervisors or co-workers typically respond? What are the immediate and delayed consequences of the behavior?	Does the learner enjoy these types of consequences? Would the consequences function as reinforcers for their behavior even if delayed?
	Immediate: Delayed:	
	Immediate: Delayed:	
	Immediate: Delayed:	
	Immediate: Delayed:	
	Immediate: Delayed:	

Appendix B

1. VSSA Arranged Situations Sample Data Sheet
2. VSSA Arranged Situations Template Data Sheet
3. VSSA Additional Behaviors Data Sheet (Opportunity)
4. VSSA Additional Behaviors Data Sheet (Interval)
5. VSSA Additional Behaviors Data Sheet (Frequency)
6. Functional Behavior Assessment Data Sheet
7. VSSA Sample Results Report Form
8. VSSA Template Results Report Form
9. VSSI Arranged Situations Template Data Sheet
10. VSSI Graphing Template (Percentage)
11. VSSI Graphing Template (Frequency)
12. VSSI Graphing Template (Rate)
13. VSSI Graphing Template (Rate-Blank)

1. VSSA Arranged Situations Sample Data Sheet

Arranged Situations Data Sheet (Sample)

Learner: _____ Date: _____ Instructor: _____ Data Collector: _____

Task Interrupted

Session #	# correct	# of opp.	%
Completes new task			
Returns to initial task/Asks			

Provided Feedback

Session #	# correct	# of opp.	%
Clear (C); Conflicting (F); Vague (V)			
Acknowledges			
Asks for clear feedback			
Confirms understanding			
Corrects mistake/complies			

Supervisor Unavailable

Session #	# correct	# of opp.	%
Returns to work area			
Begins additional task			
Seeks out supervisor			

Task Completion

Session #	# correct	# of opp.	%
Seeks out supervisor			
Makes "done" statement			
Inquires/begins new task			

Vague Instructions/Task not in Repertoire

Session #	# correct	# of opp.	%
Seeks assistance			
Makes help statement			

Materials Needed

Session #	# correct	# of opp.	%
Searches for materials			
Finds materials			
Seeks assistance			
Makes help statement			

End of Break

Session #	# correct	# of opp.	%
Resumes Work			

Notes:

Scoring: (+) correct; (-) incorrect; (N) no opportunity

2. VSSA Arranged Situations Template Data Sheet

Learner: _____ Date: _____ **Arranged Situations Data Sheet (Template)** Instructor: _____ Data Collector: _____

Situation:

Session #		# correct	# of opp.	%

Situation:

Session #		# correct	# of opp.	%

Situation:

Session #		# correct	# of opp.	%

Situation:

Session #		# correct	# of opp.	%

Situation:

Session #		# correct	# of opp.	%

Situation:

Session #		# correct	# of opp.	%

Situation:

Session #		# correct	# of opp.	%

Situation:

Session #		# correct	# of opp.	%

Scoring: (+) correct; (-) incorrect; (N) no opportunity

3. VSSA Additional Behaviors Data Sheet (Opportunity)

Learner: _____ Date: _____   **Additional Behaviors Data Sheet**   Instructor: _____   Data Collector: _____

Opportunity-Based Recording

Scoring: (+) correct; (−) incorrect; On-task (+) scored if no more than _____ minutes/seconds off task

Date						# correct	# of opp.
Opportunities or Session #							
							%

B1:

Scoring: (+) correct; (−) incorrect; On-task (+) scored if no more than _____ minutes/seconds off task

Date						# correct	# of opp.
Opportunities or Session #							
							%

B2:

Scoring: (+) correct; (−) incorrect; On-task (+) scored if no more than _____ minutes/seconds off task

Date						# correct	# of opp.
Opportunities or Session #							
							%

B3:

Scoring: (+) correct; (−) incorrect; On-task (+) scored if no more than _____ minutes/seconds off task

Date						# correct	# of opp.
Opportunities or Session #							
							%

B4:

Scoring: (+) correct; (−) incorrect; On-task (+) scored if no more than _____ minutes/seconds off task

Date						# correct	# of opp.
Opportunities or Session #							
							%

B5:

4. VSSA Additional Behaviors Data Sheet (Interval)

Learner: _____   Date: _____

Additional Behaviors
Interval Recording

Instructor: _____   Data Collector: _____

Scoring: (Y) if the behavior occurred; (N) if the behavior did not occur

Session # _____   Date _____

(Interval Length: _____)

	1	2	3	4	5	6	7	8	9	10	11	12	13	14	15	16	17	18	19	20	# Yes	# of intervals	%
B1:																							
B2:																							
B3:																							

Session # _____   Date _____

(Interval Length: _____)

	1	2	3	4	5	6	7	8	9	10	11	12	13	14	15	16	17	18	19	20	# Yes	# of intervals	%
B1:																							
B2:																							
B3:																							

Session # _____   Date _____

(Interval Length: _____)

	1	2	3	4	5	6	7	8	9	10	11	12	13	14	15	16	17	18	19	20	# Yes	# of intervals	%
B1:																							
B2:																							
B3:																							

Session # _____   Date _____

(Interval Length: _____)

	1	2	3	4	5	6	7	8	9	10	11	12	13	14	15	16	17	18	19	20	# Yes	# of intervals	%
B1:																							
B2:																							
B3:																							

5. VSSA Additional Behaviors Data Sheet (Frequency)

Learner: _____

Additional Behaviors Data Sheet   Instructor: _____   Data Collector: _____

Frequency Recording

Scoring: (/) for each occurrence of the behavior

Date/Session #/Time (min)			Total #	Total min	Rate (#/min)
B1:					
Rate (#/min):					

Date/Session #/Time (min)			Total #	Total min	Rate (#/min)
B2:					
Rate (#/min):					

Date/Session #/Time (min)			Total #	Total min	Rate (#/min)
B3:					
Rate (#/min):					

Date/Session #/Time (min)			Total #	Total min	Rate (#/min)
B4:					
Rate (#/min):					

Date/Session #/Time (min)			Total #	Total min	Rate (#/min)
B5:					
Rate (#/min):					

6. Functional Behavior Assessment Data Sheet

Learner: _____   **Functional Behavior Assessment**   Instructor: _____
Date: _____   **Data Sheet**   Data Collector: _____

Target Behavior:	Definition:

											Total # of Instances		
Immediate Antecedent	Scoring: (X) for each instance of the behavior										Attention	Escape	Tangible
Supervisor unavailable													
Ignored by others													
Provided feedback													
Task interrupted													
Coworker asks for assistance													
Given clear instruction													
Given vague instruction													
Task not in repertoire													
Materials needed													
Conversing with peer													
Denied access to items/activities													

Immediate consequence

											Attention	Escape	Tangible
Given feedback/attention													
Ignored													
Task delayed or removed													
Provided items/activities													
Provided break													
											Totals:		

If the highest number of instances of the target behavior were scored as **attention**, this indicates the learner most likely engages in the target behavior to access attention; this may be in the form of conversation, reprimands, or a reaction.

If the highest number of instances of the target behavior were scored as **escape**, this indicates the learner most likely engages in the target behavior to avoid work, get out of completing certain tasks, or get a break.

If the highest number of instances of the target behavior were scored as **tangible**, this indicates the learner most likely engages in the target behavior to gain access to an item or activity such as food, electronics, or personal items.

7. VSSA Sample Results Report Form

Learner: _____ Date: _____

VSSA Results Report (Sample)

Instructor: _____ End of Break: _____ Data Collector: _____

	Task Interrupted	Provided Feedback	Materials Needed	Vague Instructions	Task not in Repertoire	Supervisor Unavailable	End of Break	Task Completion
91-100%								
81-90%								
71-80%								
61-70%								
51-60%								
41-50%								
31-40%								
21-30%								
11-20%								
0-10%								
Opportunities								

Task Interrupted: Completes new task / Returns to initial task/Asks

Provided Feedback: Acknowledges / Asks for clear feedback / Confirms understanding / Corrects mistake/complies

Materials Needed: Searches for materials / Finds materials / Seeks assistance / Makes help statement

Vague Instructions: Seeks assistance / Makes help statement

Task not in Repertoire: Seeks assistance / Makes help statement

Supervisor Unavailable: Returns to work area / Begins additional task / Seeks out supervisor

End of Break: Resumes work

Task Completion: Seeks out supervisor / Makes "done" statement / Inquires/begin new task

Additional Behaviors

Behavior	% / # / Rate		Behavior	% / # / Rate

Inappropriate Behaviors

Behavior	% / # / Rate		Behavior	% / # / Rate

8. VSSA Template Results Report Form

VSSA Results Report (Template)

Learner: _____ Date: _____   Instructor: _____   Data Collector: _____

| | 91-100% | 81-90% | 71-80% | 61-70% | 51-60% | 41-50% | 31-40% | 21-30% | 11-20% | 0-10% | Opportunities |

Additional Appropriate Behaviors

Behavior	%/#/ Rate	Behavior	%/#/ Rate

Inappropriate Behaviors

Behavior	%/#/ Rate	Behavior	%/#/ Rate

9. VSSI Arranged Situations **Template** Data Sheet

VSSI Arranged Situations Data Sheet

Learner: _____   Instructor: _____   Data Collector: _____

Situation:

Date														
Session #														

Percentage (correct/total): _____

Situation:

Date														
Session #														

Percentage (correct/total): _____

Situation:

Date														
Session #														

Percentage (correct/total): _____

10. VSSI Graphing Template (Percentage)

VSSI Graphing Template (Percentage)

Learner: _____   Date: _____   Instructor: _____   Data Collector: _____

Arranged Situation: _____   Target: _____

Phase

| Yes 91-100% |
| 81-90% |
| 71-80% |
| 61-70% |
| 51-60% |
| 41-50% |
| 31-40% |
| 21-30% |
| 11-20% |
| No 0-10% |
| Session |

Arranged Situation: _____   Target: _____

Phase

| Yes 91-100% |
| 81-90% |
| 71-80% |
| 61-70% |
| 51-60% |
| 41-50% |
| 31-40% |
| 21-30% |
| 11-20% |
| No 0-10% |
| Session |

11. VSSI Graphing Template (Frequency)

VSSI Graphing Template (Frequency)

Learner: _____   Date: _____   Instructor: _____   Data Collector: _____

Arranged Situation: _____   Target: _____

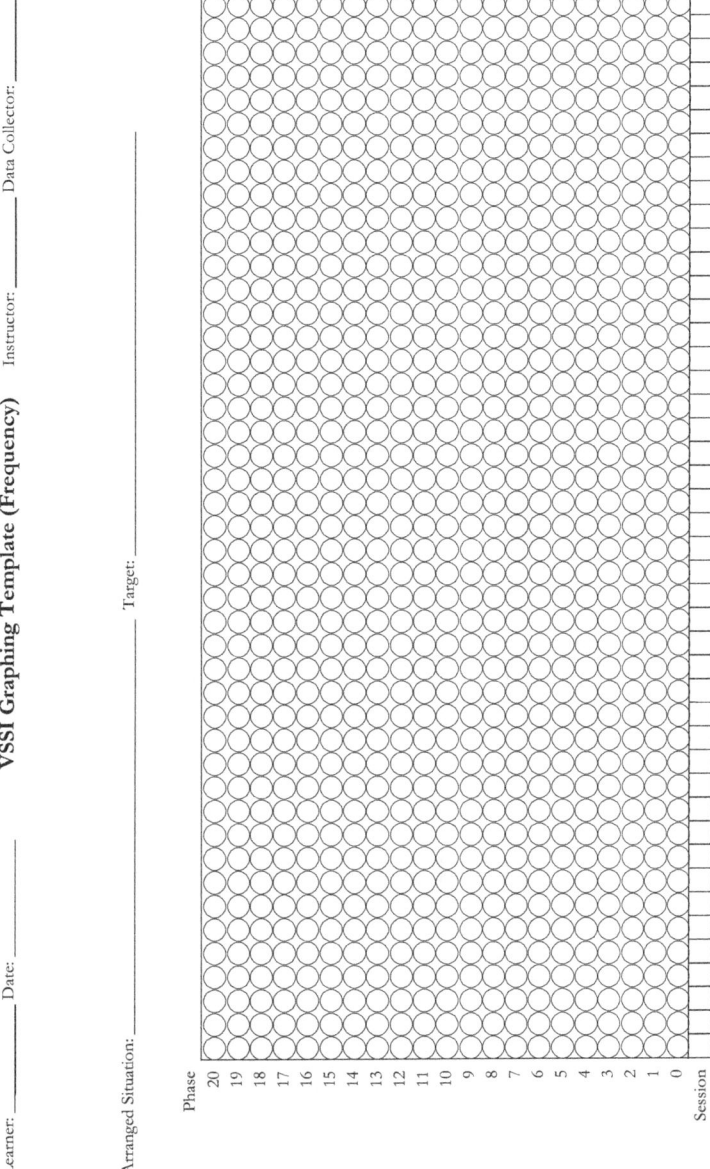

12. VSSI Graphing Template (Rate)

Learner: _____ Date: _____

VSSI Graphing Template (Rate)

Instructor: _____ Data Collector: _____

Arranged Situation: _____ Target: _____

Phase

2.0
1.9
1.8
1.7
1.6
1.5
1.4
1.3
1.2
1.1
1.0
0.9
0.8
0.7
0.6
0.5
0.4
0.3
0.2
0.1
0

Session

13. VSSI Graphing Template (Rate-Blank)

Learner: _____ Date: _____

VSSI Graphing Template (Blank-Rate)

Instructor: _____ Data Collector: _____

Arranged Situation: _____ Target: _____

Phase: _____

Rate of Behavior (Responses per Minute)

Session

Directions: along the vertical *y*-axis, fill in the units in the space provided. To determine what increments to use, estimate the highest rate of behavior and divide by 20 (the number of spaces). This will give you a rough estimate of what size increment is needed (e.g., 0.1, 0.2, 0.5, 1.0).

Example 1: if you predict the highest rate will be 2.0, you will have space to use increments of 0.1 (i.e., 0, 0.1, 0.2, 0.3).

Example 2: if you predict the highest rate will be 5.0, you will need to use larger increments such as 0.5, (i.e., 0, 0.1-0.5, 0.6-1.0, 1.1-1.5, etc.).

Index